Alcohol, Gender and Drinking Problems

Perspectives from Low and Middle Income Countries

Edited by
Isidore S. Obot & Robin Room

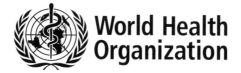

World Health Organization

Department of Mental Health and Substance Abuse, Geneva

WHO Library Cataloguing-in-Publication Data

Alcohol, gender and drinking problems: perspectives from low and middle income countries.

1. Alcohol drinking - adverse effects 2. Alcoholic intoxication - epidemiology 3. Sex factors 4. Socioeconomic factors 5. Multicenter studies 6. Developing countries I. World Health Organization II. GENACIS.

ISBN 92 4 156302 8   (NLM classification: WM 274)

Typesetting: e-BookServices.com, India
Cover design: Tushita Graphic Vision Sàrl, Geneva, Switzerland
Printed in China

CONTENTS

FOREWORD

In the year 2000 the Department of Health of the Government of Valencia, Spain, received a proposal from the Department of Mental Health and Substance Dependence (now Substance Abuse) of the World Health Organization for technical cooperation and financial support for several projects on alcohol programmes and policy. The projects suggested in the proposal included data gathering, management of alcohol problems through dissemination of brief intervention, the development of global alcohol policy initiatives, and support for technology transfer in the field of substance abuse in general.

The reason behind this request for cooperation was a recognition of the growing role of alcohol in global public health, especially in developing countries, and the need for more funding to continue some of the World Health Organization's outstanding work on alcohol. For example, though WHO projects on screening and brief intervention (SBI) in primary heath care settings had been recognized as an effective strategy in reducing harmful and hazardous alcohol consumption in several developed countries, the strategy had not been tested in developing countries. The proposal also recognized the need for dependable and comparable data on gender and alcohol issues, including differences between men and women in patterns of drinking and related problems.

Data from a variety of sources, especially WHO's Global Alcohol Database (GAD) and the annual world health reports, support the contention that alcohol indeed has become a major risk factor for disease and disability in many countries across the world. That this risk is increasing in, for example, the low-mortality developing countries of Asia and South America where alcohol is often the highest contributor to disease burden.

Considering its interest in global public health, the Valencian Government was pleased to approve the signing of a cooperative agreement with WHO in 2001 and the agreement has been renewed every year since then. The agreement focused on work in the following areas: gender and alcohol, alcohol policy, and knowledge transfer through training. One of the first activities in the agreement was a meeting of experts to discuss the implications of alcohol marketing to young people's drinking which took place in Valencia in March 2002. The product of that meeting is expected to serve as a major resource in our understanding of the role of alcohol marketing and promotion in youth drinking behaviours.

Support provided through the agreement has also been used by WHO to fund projects on brief intervention for alcohol problems in Brazil and South Africa. It has also led to this book which is the product of the gender and alcohol project in seven countries on four continents (namely,

Argentina, Costa Rica, India, Kazakhstan, Nigeria, Sri Lanka and Uganda).

I am indeed pleased to contribute the foreword to this book which publishes contributions on gender and alcohol from six of the countries funded through the Valencia-WHO cooperative agreement and two other countries. The book will go a long way in enhancing our appreciation of gender issues in alcohol research and in the management of alcohol-related problems not only in primary care but in other settings, e.g., prenatal clinics and the workplace. I am sure that the book will contribute to the development of alcohol policy and the provision of service to men and women with alcohol-related problems not only in the countries in the reports but all around the world. The Government of Valencia, through the Department of Health, is happy to be associated with WHO's commitment to reducing alcohol problems globally and will continue to support its efforts in achieving this goal.

Dr Bartolomé Pérez Gálvez

Director General, Drug Dependence
Department of Health
Autonomous Government of Valencia
Spain

PREFACE

This book presents data and addresses significant issues on gender and alcohol in eight low and middle income countries where such data are often not available. The book is a product of the multinational collaborative project on "Gender, Alcohol and Culture: an International Study" (GENACIS). GENACIS was funded by the European Commission, the U.S. National Institute on Alcoholism and Alcohol Abuse (NIAAA), the Swiss Office of Education and Science, the German Federal Ministry of Public Health, the World Health Organization, government agencies and other sources in individual countries.

The study was conceived by the International Research Group on Gender and Alcohol (IRGGA), a group of researchers affiliated with the Kettil Bruun Society for Social and Epidemiological Research on Alcohol (KBS). Beginning with a few countries in 1999, GENACIS grew to include projects in more than thirty countries and 50 researchers, all united by a common interest in seeking greater understanding of gender and alcohol issues.

GENACIS uses a centralized data analysis and standardized measures to assess the differences between men and women within and across cultures in the following areas:

- patterns and contexts of drinking;
- prevalence of alcohol problems;
- the experience of drinking-related violence in close relationships;
- how social inequalities and social roles influence drinking and heavy alcohol consumption;
- the relationship of societal-level factors (e.g., gender equality, drinking culture norms) to drinking and alcohol-related problems.

The study grew out of earlier projects in Europe and the U.S. and seeks to clarify further the factors associated with men's and women's drinking and alcohol-related problems.

GENACIS is truly an international project; participating countries are drawn from all parts of the world, especially from countries where harmful use of alcohol poses a threat to public health and social welfare. Funding provided to WHO by the Government of Valencia, Spain, made it possible for countries in low and middle income countries to participate in the project. These countries are Argentina, Costa Rica, India, Kazakhstan, Nigeria, Sri Lanka and Uganda. There are also ongoing WHO-funded projects in three countries in the region of the Americas.

The papers published in this book report data from six of these countries and from two other countries (Brazil and Mexico) participating in GENACIS. Each paper addresses a particular issue of relevance to the country and provides a general overview of drinking and alcohol problems.

All papers evolved through a series of revisions after consultations with and reviews by a team of experts associated with the project. These experts and lead authors participated in group discussions held in Berlin, Krakow, and Helsinki during GENACIS steering committee meetings or the annual conference of the Kettil Bruun Society.

GENACIS is one of several projects on alcohol by the Department of Mental Health and Substance Abuse that are designed to enhance our understanding of alcohol problems and provide the basis for effective interventions. This product from the GENACIS project will serve as a valuable resource to researchers, service providers, policy-makers, students and all those engaged in work on alcohol and public health, and contribute to shaping a global response to the harmful consequences of alcohol.

Dr Benedetto Saraceno
Director
Department of Mental Health and Substance Abuse

ACKNOWLEDGEMENTS

The preparation and publication of this book would not have been possible without the generous financial contribution of the Autonomous Government of Valencia, Spain, to the World Health Organization for projects on Alcohol and Public Health. This support started in 2001 with a grant for work in three related areas — gender and alcohol, screening and brief intervention for alcohol problems, and alcohol policy. The grant made it possible for WHO to sponsor the participation of researchers from low and middle income countries in the multinational project on Gender, Alcohol and Culture: an International Study (GENACIS).

Special thanks are due to Dr Bartolomé Pérez Gálvez, Director General for Drug Dependence, Department of Health, Autonomous Government of Valencia, for his exceptional commitment to the GENACIS project and his overall interest in working with WHO to reduce alcohol related problems in developing countries. Several staff of the Department of Health in Valencia, especially Dr José Martinez-Raga, also contributed in various ways to the success of the projects funded by their office.

The participation of contributors in project meetings (in Berlin, Krakow and Helsinki) was made possible by grants from the U.S. National Institute on Alcohol Abuse and Alcoholism/National Institutes of Health (R01AA04610 and R21AA12941), and the European Union's Fifth Framework Research Programme (contract QLG4-CT-2001-01496). Grateful thanks are due to the principal investigators in these grants (Sharon Wilsnack and Kim Bloomfield, respectively), and to Arlinda Kristjanson, Stephanie Kramer, and Friedericke Froehner for facilitating the participation of contributors in these meetings in various ways.

Richard Wilsnack and Sharon Wilsnack reviewed the papers in this volume and provided guidance to contributors during the preparation of the manuscripts, and Gerhard Gmel provided advice on data management and statistical analysis. Their contributions greatly enhanced the quality of the papers published in this volume.

The WHO-GENACIS project was initiated by Maristela Monteiro and continued under the coordination of Vladimir Poznyak. Both of them provided the support and encouragement needed at different stages of the project, including the publication of this book.

Tess Narciso and Mylene Schreiber provided invaluable secretarial support for all activities related to the WHO/GENACIS project. Isidore Obot had overall responsibility for the implementation of the project in the seven WHO funded countries and represented WHO in the steering committee of the multinational research initiative.

CHAPTER 1

WHY STUDY GENDER, ALCOHOL AND CULTURE?

RICHARD W. WILSNACK, SHARON C. WILSNACK & ISIDORE S. OBOT

INTRODUCTION

Alcoholic beverages have been a part of social life for millennia, yet societies have always found it difficult to understand or restrain their use. A central theme of this book is that to better understand alcohol consumption and its consequences, we need to better understand social and cultural influences on the differences between men and women. That theme deserves careful and detailed attention for several reasons.

First, compared with women throughout the world, men are more likely to drink, consume more alcohol, and cause more problems by doing so. This gender gap is one of the few universal gender differences in human social behavior. It is evident in all areas of the world (Almeida-Filho et al., 2004; Degenhardt et al., 1997; McKee et al., 2000; Perdrix et al., 1999; Rijken, Velema, & Dijkstra, 1998; Sieri et al., 2002), in drinking versus abstinence (Mohan, Chopra, & Sethi, 2002; Peltzer, 2002), in heavy drinking and intoxication (Gmel, Rehm, & Kuntsche, 2003; Higuchi et al., 1994; Siegfried et al., 2001), and in alcohol use disorders (Jhingan et al., 2003; Kebede & Alem, 1999; Yamamoto et al., 1993). The gender gap has varied but persisted for a long time, at least in European history (Martin, 2001; Plant, 1997; Sandmaier, 1980; Warner, 1997) and in the traditions of many pre-industrial societies elsewhere (Child, Barry, & Bacon, 1965; Seale et al., 2002; Suggs, 2001; Willis, 2001).

Research has suggested several possible reasons why universal gender differences in drinking behavior might arise. For example, if women have lower rates of gastric metabolism of alcohol than men (Baraona et al., 2001; Frezza et al., 1990; Thomasson, 1995) or smaller volumes of body water in which alcohol is distributed (Mirand & Welte, 1994; York & Welte, 1994), women may need to consume less alcohol than men to derive the same effects. Or, women may be more likely than men to experience unpleasant acute effects from alcohol (such as hangover symptoms) (Slutske et al., 1995, 2003), or may not enjoy risky and poorly controlled behavioral effects of alcohol as much as men (Hill & Chow, 2002; Rosenblitt et al., 2001; Spigner, Hawkins, & Lorens, 1993), characteristics which might inhibit women's drinking. However, despite the universality of gender differences in drinking behavior, the size of gender differences has varied greatly in different societies, historical eras, and drinking patterns; and neither the universality nor the variability of those gender differences has yet been adequately explained (Graham et al., 1998; Watten, 1997; R. Wilsnack et al., 2000).

A second important reason to study how gender and alcohol interact is that some of the gender differences in drinking, and much of the variation in such gender differences, are cultural. Societies have long used alcohol consumption and its effects as important ways to differentiate, symbolize, and regulate gender roles (Joffe, 1998; Warner, 1997). Differences in normative drinking patterns help reveal to what extent societies differentiate gender roles, for example, by making drinking behavior a demonstration of masculinity (Campbell, 2000; Driessen, 1992; MacDonald, 1994; Roberts, 2004; Suggs, 1996) or by forbidding women to drink as a symbol of subservience or to prevent sexual autonomy (Martin, 2001; Nicolaides, 1996; Willis, 1999). Better understanding of how men's and women's drinking patterns differ is thus an important key to answering broader questions of how and why societies try to get women and men to behave differently (Gefou-Madianou, 1992; MacDonald, 1994; Murdock, 2001; Wilsnack & Wilsnack, 1997).

In recent decades there has been increased concern about drinking behavior as an aspect of gender roles, because in some societies gender differences in drinking behavior have grown smaller. A common hypothesis about such *convergence* in drinking patterns is that increased opportunities for women to perform traditionally male roles (particularly in the workforce) have also enabled and encouraged women to increase their drinking, with more adverse consequences (Bergmark, 2004; Bloomfield et al., 2001). Consistent with this hypothesis, where convergence has occurred, it has usually been most evident among adolescents or young adults (Grant et al., 2004; McPherson, Casswell, & Pledger, 2004; Mercer & Khavari, 1990; Plant et al., 1999). However, convergence has not always occurred where it might be expected (Bloomfield et al., 2001; Neve et al., 1996; Serdula et al., 2004; Williams, 1998); it may occur for some aspects of drinking behavior but not others (Grant et al., 2004; Malyutina et al., 2004); it may sometimes occur because men are drinking less instead of women drinking more (Bergmark, 2004; O'Brien et al., 2001; Osler et al., 2001); and it is not always related to women's nontraditional roles (Malyutina et al., 2004; Neve et al, 1996). If social influences on women's and men's drinking are likely to be historically and culturally complex, better cross-cultural research on gender and drinking over longer periods of time may be essential to avoid oversimplified conclusions about effects of changes in women's and men's roles.

A third important reason to study how gender affects alcohol use is that false assumptions about male or female drinking may adversely affect how societies identify and try to control alcohol-related problems. If heavy drinking is associated with displays of masculinity or male camaraderie, this may encourage male drinkers to deny or minimize problems resulting from their drinking, or to regard drunken behavior as normal or permissible (Capraro, 2000; Nayak, 2003; Nghe, Mahalik, & Lowe, 2003), even when it leads to violence (Graham & Wells, 2003; Hunt & Laidler, 2001; Tomsen, 1997). On the other hand, assumptions that women do not drink heavily may lead to women's drinking problems being underestimated or overlooked (for example, by physicians; Brienza & Stein, 2002; Denny et al., 2003; Malet et al. 2003; Svikis & Reid-Quinones, 2003). However, when women's alcohol abuse or dependence becomes conspicuous, it has often provoked social outrage and the use of punishment or coercion to try to stop such behavior (Blume, 1997; McLaughlin, 1991; Sandmaier, 1980), most recently by taking custody of children (Dolgin, 1991; Nishimoto & Roberts, 2001) or by forcing alcohol-abusing women to be hospitalized or incarcerated if pregnant (Abel & Kruger, 2002; DeVille & Kopelman, 1998). Better understanding of gender stereotypes about both men's and women's drinking is essential to reduce the negative effects such stereotypes may have on treatment and prevention of alcohol-related problems.

THEORETICAL ISSUES: WHICH GENDER DIFFERENCES?

Efforts to understand and explain gender differences in drinking behavior must deal with several theoretical questions. The first question is, which gender differences are important to explain? Nearly all studies that measure lifetime abstinence from alcohol find that such abstinence is much more common among women than among men (e.g., Assanangkornchai, Pinkaew, & Apakupakul, 2003; Beals et al., 2003; Caraveo- Anduaga et al., 1999; Meyer et al., 2000; Vahtera et al., 2002; Wilsnack et al., 2000; Zhang et al., 2004). Table 1 shows the total consumption of alcohol (in litres of absolute alcohol), average consumption per drinker, and the proportions of male and female current drinkers in fourteen World Health Organization subregional groupings (current drinkers are those who had an alcoholic drink in the last 12 months). The subregions are defined on the basis of child and adult mortality rates where, for example, A represents countries with very low child and very low adult mortality and E means that countries in that group have high rates of child mortality and very high adult mortality (Ezzati, 2002). It is clear from the table that in all regions more males than females consume alcohol, but in some regions the differences are not as marked as in others (WHO, 2004a).

Gender ratios (male/female) for drinking in the past 12 months or for being a former drinker are generally larger than gender ratios for lifetime abstinence, and in most surveys the gender ratios (male/female) increase progressively from lifetime abstainers to former drinkers to

3

TABLE 1. **Adult alcohol consumption and male-female consumption in 14 WHO sub-regions, 2000**

WHO sub-region	Total consumption (litres of absolute alcohol)	Consumption per drinker	% Male current drinkers	% Female current drinkers
Africa D (e.g., Nigeria, Algeria)	4.9	13.3	47	27
Africa E (e.g., Ethiopía, South Africa)	7.1	16.6	55	30
Americas A (Canada, Cuba, USA)	9.3	14.3	73	58
Americas B (e.g., Brazil, Mexico)	9.0	14.1	75	53
Americas D (e.g., Bolivia, Peru)	5.1	7.6	74	60
Eastern Mediterranean B (e.g., Iran, Saudi Arabia)	1.3	11.0	18	4
Eastern Mediterranean D (e.g., Afghanistan, Pakistan)	0.6	6.0	17	1
Europe A (e.g., Germany, France, UK)	12.9	15.1	90	81
Europe B (e.g., Bulgaria, Poland, Turkey)	8.3	13.4	72	52
Europe C (e.g., Russian Federation, Ukraine	13.9	16.5	89	81
Southeast Asia B (e.g., Indonesia, Thailand)	3.1	13.7	35	9
Southeast Asia D (e.g., Bangladesh, India)	2.0	12.9	26	4
Western Pacific A (e.g., Australia, Japan)	8.5	10.4	87	77
Western Pacific B (e.g., China, Philippines, Vietnam)	5.0	8.8	84	30

Source: World Health Organization, 2004a

current drinkers (e.g., Assanangkornchai et al., 2003; Meyer et al., 2000; Rehm, Greenfield, & Rogers, 2001; Welty et al., 1995; Zhang et al., 2004).

At the other extreme, surveys in many different populations consistently find that men are more than twice as likely as women to report heavy episodic drinking (or "binge" drinking, of at least 60 grams of ethanol in a day) (e.g., Janghorbani et al., 2003; Malyutina et al., 2001; Miller et al, 2004; Neumark, Rahav, & Jaffe, 2003; Welte et al., 1995;

Wilsnack et al., 2000). Men are also consistently more than twice as likely as women to report chronic heavy drinking (at mean intake thresholds varying from 40 to 80 grams of ethanol per day) (e.g., de Lima et al., 2003; Hansagi et al., 1995; Meyer et al., 2000; San Jose et al., 2001; Vahtera et al., 2002). Recurrent alcohol intoxication is much more prevalent and more frequent among men than among women (Hao et al., 2004; Makela et al, 2001; Rehm et al., 2001). However, gender gaps in chronic or episodic heavy drinking may be smaller among late adolescents or university students (Dawson et al., 2004; Kuo et al., 2002; McPherson et al., 2004; Windle, 2003). As shown in Table 2, gender gaps in the prevalence of heavy episodic drinking have become small or nonexistent in some European countries (such as Ireland, Norway and the United Kingdom), but also in some developing countries (such as Nigeria and Mexico) (WHO, 2004a).

Consistent with gender differences in heavy drinking, surveys in many countries find that men are more than twice as likely as women to have alcohol use disorders. Men are much more likely than women to report diagnosable alcohol abuse, either currently (e.g., Bijl et al., 2002; Dawson, Grant, & Stinson, 2004; Hao et al., 2004; Kringlen, Torgersen, & Cramer, 2001; Yamamoto et al., 1993) or as a lifetime experience (Kawakami et al., 2004; Meyer et al., 2000). Men are also much more likely than women to report diagnosable alcohol dependence, currently (e.g., Bijl et al., 2002; Hao et al., 2004; Hasin & Grant, 2004; Kawakami et al, 2004; Spicer et al., 2003) or as a lifetime experience (Dawson & Grant, 1998; Heath et al., 1997; Kawakami et al. 2004; Meyer et al, 2000). In surveys administering the Alcohol Use Disorders Identification Test

TABLE 2. **Male-female differences in heavy episodic drinking among young people in selected countries**

Country	Year	Total (%)	Male (%)	Female (%)	Age group
Australia	2001	10.7	9.6	11.8	14-19
Canada	2000-2001	15.3	26.3	5.2	15-19
China	2000-2001	1.3	2.5	0.0	15-19
Finland	1999	18.0	21.0	15.0	15-16
France	1999	12.0	16.0	7.0	15-16
Hungary	2003	27.5	39.2	22.2	15-16
Ireland	1999	31.0	32.0	32.0	15-16
India	2000-2001	0.5	1.2	0.0	15-19
Mexico	2000-2001	2.5	0.8	1.5	15-19
Nigeria	2000-2001	1.2	1.0	1.3	15-19
Norway	2003	15.0	17.0	14.0	15-16
UK	1999	30.0	33.0	27.0	15-16
USA	2002	10.7	11.4	9.9	12-17

Source: World Health Organization, 2004a

(AUDIT), men are consistently more than twice as likely as women to receive scores of 8 or more, a conventional threshold for identifying probable alcohol use disorders (Assanangkornchai et al., 2003; Bergman & Kallmen, 2002; Mendoza-Sassi & Beria, 2003; Morales-Garcia et al., 2002; Singleton et al., 2003). In addition, there is consistent evidence that deaths and poisoning attributable to alcohol are much more likely to occur among men than among women (Ramstedt, 2002; Rivara et al., 2004; Yoon et al., 2003).

One way of comparing the extent of problems experienced by men and women because of their drinking is through the World Health Organization Comparative Risk Assessment (CRA). The CRA is part of the Global Burden of Disease (GBD) study and focuses on the impact of 26 identified risk factors on the burden of disease. Because GBD data do not include social harms caused by alcohol, the data reported in table 3 are underestimates of alcohol's total burden on society. However, data reported in the table support the overall finding that many health conditions associated with harmful and hazardous consumption of alcohol are more prevalent among men than women. The numbers in the table refer to disability adjusted life years (DALYs), a summary measure which combines years of life lost to premature death and years lived with disability from diseases and injuries. One DALY is equivalent to the loss of one healthy life year (WHO, 2002). In summary, Table 3 shows that in 2000 alcohol was responsible for 1.3% of DALYs in women and 6.5% in men. Indeed, alcohol ranks fourth (and tobacco fifth at 4.1%) among 20 leading risk factors for death and disability globally (Rehm et al., 2003). In low-mortality developing countries, alcohol is the leading risk factor for burden of disease, accounting for 6.2% of DALYs (WHO, 2002). For example, in this category of countries in the Americas (represented in this book by Argentina, Brazil, Costa Rica, and Mexico), 11.4% of DALYs are attributable to alcohol.

Unfortunately, research on differences in how men and women drink (or abstain) still has major limitations. Many epidemiological studies do not distinguish lifetime abstainers from former drinkers, despite the importance of doing so for evaluating health effects of alcohol consumption (Dawson, 2003; Fagrell et al., 1999). Threshold levels for heavy episodic drinking differ between studies and often differ categorically for men and women (i.e., not based on characteristics of individual drinkers), making it difficult to interpret comparisons of heavy drinking prevalence between genders and across studies. Many studies estimate the prevalence of heavy drinking (and alcohol disorders) in the total population but not among current drinkers, so apparent gender differences are inflated by gender differences in abstinence. Studies comparing men's and women's abstinence or drinking often do not provide age-specific or age-standardized data, obscuring how age may affect how women and men abstain, drink, or stop drinking. Finally, much of the research heretofore

6

TABLE 3. Global burden of disease in 2000 attributable to alcohol according to major disease categories (DALYs in 000s)

Disease or Injury	Female	Male	Total
Conditions arising during the perinatal period	55	68	123
Malignant neoplasm	1021	3180	4201
Neuro-psychiatric conditions	3814	18 090	21 904
Cardiovascular diseases	-428	4411	3983
Other non-communicable diseases (diabetes, liver cirrhosis)	860	3695	4555
Unintentional injuries	2487	14 008	16 495
Intentional injuries	1117	5945	7062
Alcohol-related disease burden all causes (DALYs)	8926	49 397	58 323
All DALYs	693 911	761 562	1 455 473
% of all DALYs that can be attributable to alcohol	1.3	6.5	4.0

Source: Rehm et al. (2003)

on gender and drinking has been confined to Europe and North America. The studies reported in the chapters to follow make considerable progress toward overcoming many of these limitations.

THEORETICAL ISSUES: EXPLAINING GENDER INFLUENCES ON DRINKING

As noted above, the apparently universal differences in how women and men consume alcohol suggest that to some extent there may be biological bases for these differences. However, the enormous cross-cultural variation in the size of the gaps between men's and women's drinking require other more cultural and social-structural explanations. Research thus far has suggested four categories of possible sociocultural reasons why men's and women's drinking patterns remain dissimilar: power, sex, risks, and responsibilities.

Power. The most common hypotheses to explain why men and women differ in their drinking behavior argue that alcohol consumption both symbolizes and enhances men's greater power relative to women (McClelland et al., 1972). Alcohol consumption, particularly in large quantities, has been an emblem of male superiority, a privilege that men have often reserved for themselves and denied to women (Martin, 2001; Nicolaides, 1996; Purcell, 1994; Suggs, 1996, 2001; Wang et al., 1992; Willis, 1999). Alcohol consumption in all-male groups may affirm the privileged status of being a man rather than a woman (Campbell, 2000;

Hunt & Laidler, 2001; Nghe et al., 2003, Taillon, 2002), and the ability to consume large amounts of alcohol without apparent impairment may help to demonstrate that the drinker is manly (Neff, Prihoda, & Hoppe, 1991; Roberts, 2004). Because drinking historically has been a male privilege, increases in women's drinking have been linked to social changes that allow women to perform other roles once reserved for men (Bergmark, 2004; Kubicka, Csemy, & Kozeny, 1995; McPherson et al., 2004; Takano, Nakamura, & Watanabe, 1996). However, failures to find simple or consistent effects of paid employment on women's drinking in Europe and North America (Ames & Rebhun, 1996; Lahelma, Kangas, & Manderbacka, 1995; Neve et al., 1996; Romelsjo & Lundberg, 1996; Wilsnack & Wilsnack, 1992) suggest that increased autonomy and opportunities to perform traditionally male roles have not been enough to cause women to drink the way that men do.

Alcohol may seem to enhance power over others by facilitating aggressive behavior, Much research, particularly in laboratory studies of college students, has established that drinking leads to increased aggression toward other people, more by men than by women (Bushman, 1997; Harford, Wechsler, & Muthen, 2003; Scott, Schafer, & Greenfield, 1999). However, this effect of alcohol depends to some degree on personal characteristics of male drinkers (Parrott & Giancola, 2004; Giancola, 2003), expectations that alcohol makes people aggressive (Giancola, 2002; Quigley, Corbett, & Tedeschi, 2002), and environments that facilitate hostile encounters (Graham, West, & Wells, 2000). In short, men who may want to bully or assault other people learn that alcohol can help them do this in certain circumstances. In particular, heavy drinking is likely to be a context or prelude for male violence against women, either in attacks on intimate partners (Fals-Stewart, 2003; Graham, Plant, & Plant, 2004; O'Leary & Schumacher, 2003; Wells & Graham, 2003; White & Chen, 2002) or more generally in sexual assaults (Abbey, 2002; Abbey et al., 2003; Testa, 2002). While greater aggressiveness toward women could encourage more than discourage men's drinking, it is not clear that alcohol's effects on men's aggression would be a disincentive for women's drinking, particularly if women use alcohol not so much to aid their own aggression as to help them cope with the emotional consequences of being attacked (Corbin et al., 2001; Kilpatrick et al., 1997; Testa & Leonard, 2001; Testa, Livingston, & Leonard, 2003).

Sex. Both men and women may be motivated to drink by expectations that alcohol will enhance their sexual performance and enjoyment (or will make it easier for them to engage in sexual activity) (Demmel & Hagen, 2004; MacLatchy-Gaudet & Stewart, 2001; MacQueen et al., 1996; S. Wilsnack et al., 1997). These expectations may be more influential for men than women (Anderson & Mathieu, 1996; Morr & Mongeau, 2004; Wall, Hinson, & McKee, 1998), but such comparisons are based mainly on U. S. college students. However, fears that alcohol makes women sexually more active and indiscriminate, or makes women more open to sexual advances, have contributed to policies aimed to prevent or minimize women's drinking (McLaughlin, 1991; Nicolaides, 1996; Sandmaier, 1980; West, 1997), and have reinforced social disapproval of women's drinking (Leigh, 1995; Roberts, 2004). Hypothetically, women have been socially influenced to drink less than men partly as a way to restrain women's sexual behavior. However, to the extent that women are aware that their drinking may increase their risks of or vulnerability to male sexual aggression (Abbey, 2002; Abbey et al., 2004; Testa, Vanzile-Tamsen, & Livingston, 2004), this might also be an incentive for some women to limit their own drinking relative to men.

Risks. A third theoretical approach would argue that men drink more than women do because men are generally more willing or motivated to take risks than women are (Byrnes, Miller, & Schafer, 1999; LaGrange & Silverman, 1999; Weber, Blais, & Betz, 2002). Gender differences in risk-taking may result from many possible causes: that men find risk-taking more inherently rewarding (exciting) than women do, that risk-taking is an important part of demonstrating masculinity (but not femininity), or that women perceive and/or avoid risks more than men do (Campbell, Muncer, & Bibel, 2001; Eckel & Grossman, 2002; Fetchenhauer & Rohde, 2002; Hartog, Ferrer-Carabonell, & Jonker, 2002; Zaleskiewicz, 2001) . Alcohol consumption (especially in large quantities) may not only be a form of risk-taking, but may chemically make it easier for men to take other risks (that women would be less likely to take, such as in aggressive behavior). Evidence suggests that gender differences in risk-perception or risk-taking propensity affect drinking behavior (Engwall, Hunter, & Steinberg, 2004; Spigner, Hawkins, & Loren, 1993; Zuckerman & Kuhlman, 2000), but that the risk-taking effects may be greatest in late adolescence and early adulthood, before men assume marital and parental roles (Byrnes et al., 1999; Hill & Chow, 2002), and/or among men whose masculinity is threatened in other areas of life (Courtenay, 2000). If men and women are likely to differ more at higher levels of risk-taking (Hirschberger et al., 2002), this would be consistent with the greater gender differences in the heaviest and most hazardous drinking patterns, as noted above.

Responsibilities. A fourth theoretical theme in research on gender and drinking is that men's and women's drinking are differently affected by social responsibilities. On the one hand, men may be more likely to drink heavily because drinking either helps them ignore responsibilities (particularly domestic roles) or demonstrates their immunity to role obligations (Armeli et al., 2000; Hammill, 2001; Magazine, 2004). On the other hand, greater role responsibilities, particularly at home, may cause women (more than men) to limit their drinking (Ahlstrom, Bloomfield, & Knibbe, 2001; Neve et al., 1996; Schulenberg et al., 2000; Shore, 1997; Thundal, Granbom, & Allebeck, 1999), perhaps because drinking might impair their role performance, or because women with more role responsibilities are subject to greater social surveillance (Wilsnack & Cheloha, 1987). However, inhibiting effects of multiple role responsibilities on women's drinking have not been consistent across cultures or across drinking patterns (Gmel et al., 2000; Hajema & Knibbe, 1998), and may be overridden by effects of conflicts and other distress women experience from their combined family and work roles (Frone, 1999; Grzywacz & Marks, 2000; Koopman et al., 2003; Parker & Harford, 1992). The most that can be argued at this point is that in some social contexts, domestic role obligations affect men's and women's drinking differently, in ways that tend to maintain and magnify gender gaps in drinking behavior.

Summary. These four theoretical reasons for gender differences in drinking behavior may occur together, so it is possible that combinations of these reasons will be sufficient to maintain gender differences in drinking in any given culture and historical era. Note also that the four possible ways to explain gender differences may be relevant to individuals, to groups of individuals (such as in all-male drinking), and to larger societies and cultures. One possible inference is that male drinking behavior is most likely to be extreme or problematic, and gender differences in drinking behavior are likely to be greatest, where individuals, groups, or societies give the greatest value and importance to male dominance, sexual assertiveness, risk-taking, and avoidance of (domestic) responsibilities. The chief limitation of such a male-centered perspective is that it may not be helpful for explaining why some women drink in hazardous or harmful ways. It is possible that some of women's drinking patterns and problems may result from the same factors that encourage men's drinking (Lundahl et al., 1997; Wall, McKee, & Hinson, 2000; Williams & Ricciardelli, 1996) , but a growing body of research suggests that we will have to find other explanations for women's drinking that are more important for women than for men, e.g., in terms of alcohol's effects or expected benefits either to facilitate interpersonal relationships or to cope with the pains of lacking or losing such relationships (Covington & Surrey, 1997; Laitinen, Ek, & Sovio, 2002; Makela & Mustonen, 2000; McKee et al., 1998; Skaff, Finney, & Moos, 1999; Thundal et al., 1999). Among its many contributions, the research in the subsequent chapters may help to clarify what kinds of social and cultural influences may encourage women's drinking more than men's, and thus may reduce the size of the gender gap.

STUDYING GENDER, ALCOHOL AND CULTURE IN EIGHT COUNTRIES

The chapters that follow are reports based on data from the project on Gender, Alcohol and Culture: an International Study (GENACIS) conducted in eight countries in Africa, Asia and Latin America. GENACIS was initiated by an international group of alcohol researchers to carry out gender comparisons within countries and cross-nationally on patterns of drinking and the prevalence of alcohol-related problems. The study also assesses the individual and societal level factors that are associated with men's and women's drinking and drinking problems. More than 30 countries have participated in the project. Table 4 shows the countries from which data are reported in the book and highlights the diversity and some similarities in the demographic characteristics of these countries.

Four of these countries have very large populations, while the populations of others are of low to medium size. Four of the countries are in the Americas (Argentina, Brazil, Costa Rica, and Mexico), two in South East Asia (India and Sri Lanka), and two in Africa (Nigeria and Uganda). Though all are from what is generally known as the developing world, they range in economic standing from low to middle income countries, and include countries with high and low mortality rates. In terms of human development, three are ranked as high, three medium and two as low on the human development index (HDI), and there is a close similarity in rankings for HDI and gender-related development (GDI). Two of the countries with the highest HDI (Argentina and Costa Rica) are also the ones with the highest literacy rates, while Nigeria and Uganda are the lowest on both dimensions. More than half of adult females in these countries abstain from alcohol (with a range of 55% in Mexico to nearly 93% in Sri Lanka), except in Argentina where less than a quarter of the women and 7.5% of men are abstainers.

Each contribution in this book begins with a broad overview of the alcohol situation in the country, including responses to alcohol related problems. Some of the papers address several aspects of drinking, including patterns of consumption and the social and health consequences of drinking (Sri Lanka and Uganda), while others focus on social problems (Argentina and Costa Rica). One paper assesses the differences in drinking patterns between men and women (Mexico) and another compares the different contexts in which men and women drink (Nigeria). Two of the contributions (India and Mexico) focus solely on women and aim to shed more light on drinking patterns and alcohol problems among women in these countries.

These reports provide much needed data on alcohol and gender from countries where such data are often not available. They also improve our understanding of the social and cultural influences that have increased or reduced gender differences in alcohol consumption and problems, and that have led some individuals (such as women with drinking problems) to depart from gender norms or stereotypes. In an era on increasingly global marketing of alcoholic beverages, the insights from these reports are important and timely.

TABLE 4. Social characteristics and alcohol abstention in 8 GENACIS countries

Country	WHO mortality sub-stratum	Population ('000)	Annual growth rate (%) 1992-2002	Life expectancy at birth 2002 (years), M/F	Adult literacy, 2002 (%, F/M)	HDI/GDI ranks, 2002*	Expenditure on health as % of GDP, 2001	Percentage of current abstainers	
								M	F
Argentina	AMR B	37 981	1.3	70.8/78.1	97/97	34/36	9.5	7.5	23.2
Brazil	AMR B	176 257	1.4	65.7/72.3	86.5/86.2	72/60	7.6	40.0	60.5
Costa Rica	AMR B	4 094	2.4	74.8/79.5	95.9/95.7	45/44	7.2	45.0	75.0
India	SEAR D	1 049 549	1.8	60.1/62	46.4/69.0	127/103	5.1	67.1	89.3
Mexico	AMR B	101 965	1.7	71.7/76.9	88.7/92.6	53/50	6.1	22.4	55.0
Nigeria	AFR D	120 911	2.8	48/49.6	59.4/74.4	151/122	3.4	51.3	89.6
Sri Lanka	SEAR B	18 910	0.9	67.2/74.3	89.6/94.7	96/73	3.6	41.4	92.9
Uganda	AFR D	25 004	3.0	47.9/50.8	59.2/78.8	146/113	5.9	48.2	60.3

Note: *HDI = human development index; GDI = gender-related development index. Based on rankings of 177 countries, from 1 (highest) to 177 (lowest) on these measures.

Sources: The World Health Report 2004 (WHO, 2004b); *Global Status Report on Alcohol 2004* (WHO, 2004a); *Human Development Report* (Oxford University Press, 2004).

REFERENCES

Abbey, A. (2002). Alcohol-related sexual assault: A common problem of college students. *Journal of Studies on Alcohol*, **Supplement 14**, 118-128.

Abbey, A., Clinton-Sherrod, A. M., McAuslan, P., Zawacki, T., & Buck, P. O. (2003). The relationship between the quantity of alcohol consumed and the severity of sexual assaults committed by college men. *Journal of Interpersonal Violence*, **18**, 813-833.

Abbey, A., Zawacki, T., Buck, P. O., Clinton, A. M., & McAuslan, P. (2004). Sexual assault and alcohol consumption: What do we know about their relationship and what types of research are still needed? *Aggression and Violent Behavior*, **9**, 271-303.

Abel, E. L., & Kruger, M. (2002). Physician attitudes concerning legal coercion of pregnant alcohol and drug abusers. *American Journal of Obstetrics and Gynecology*, **186**, 768-772.

Ahlström, S., Bloomfield, K., & Knibbe, R. (2001). Gender differences in drinking patterns in nine European countries: Descriptive findings. *Substance Abuse*, **22**, 69-85.

Almeida-Filho, N., Lessa, I., Magalhaes, L., Araujo, M. J., Aquino, E. A., Kawachi, I., & James, S. A. (2004). Alcohol drinking patterns by gender, ethnicity, and social class in Bahia, *Brazil. Revista de Saude Publica*, **38**, 45-54.

Ames, G. M., & Rebhun, L. A. (1996). Women, alcohol and work: Interactions of gender, ethnicity and occupational culture. *Social Science and Medicine*, **43**, 1649-1663.

Anderson, P. B., & Mathieu, D. A. (1996). College students' high risk sexual behavior following alcohol consumption. *Journal of Sex and Marital Therapy*, **22**, 259-264.

Armeli, S., Carney, M. A., Tennen, H., Affleck, G., & O'Neil, T. P. (2000). Stress and alcohol use: A daily process examination of the stressor vulnerability model. *Journal of Personality and Social Psychology*, **78**, 979-994.

Assanangkornchai, S., Pinkaew, P., & Apakupakul, N. (2003). Prevalence of hazardous-harmful drinking in a southern Thai community. *Drug and Alcohol Review*, **22**, 287-293.

Baraona, E., Abittan, C. S., Dohmen, K., Moretti, M., Pozzato, G., Chayes, Z. W., Schaefer, C., & Lieber, C. S. (2001). Gender differences in pharmacokinetics of alcohol. *Alcoholism: Clinical and Experimental Research*, **25**, 502-507.

Beals, J., Spicer, P., Mitchell, C. M., Novins, D. K., Manson, S. M., et al. (2003). Racial disparities in alcohol use: Comparison of two American Indian reservation populations with national data. *American Journal of Public Health*, **93**, 1683-1688.

Bergman, H., & Kallmén, H. (2002). Alcohol use among Swedes and a psychometric evaluation of the Alcohol Use Disorders Identification Test. *Alcohol and Alcoholism*, **37**, 245-251.

Bergmark, K. H. (2004). Gender roles, family, and drinking: Women at the crossroad of drinking cultures. *Journal of Family History*, **29**, 293-307.

Bijl, R. V., de Graaf, R., Ravelli, A., Smit, F., & Vollebergh, W. A. M. (2002). Gender and age specific first incidence of DSM III R psychiatric disorders in the general population: Results from the Netherlands Mental Health Survey and Incidence Study (NEMESIS). *Social Psychiatry and Psychiatric Epidemiology*, **37**, 372-379.

Bloomfield, K., Gmel, G., Neve, R., & Mustonen, H. (2001). Investigating gender convergence in alcohol consumption in Finland, Germany, The Netherlands, and Switzerland: A repeated survey analysis. *Substance Abuse*, **22**, 39-53.

Blume, S. B. (1997). Women and alcohol: Issues in social policy. In R. W. Wilsnack & S. C. Wilsnack (Eds.), *Gender and Alcohol: Individual and Social Perspectives* (pp. 462-489). New Brunswick, NJ: Rutgers Center of Alcohol Studies.

Brienza, R. S., & Stein, M. D. (2002). Alcohol use disorders in primary care: Do gender-specific differences exist? *Journal of General Internal Medicine*, **17**, 387-397.

Bushman, B. J. (1997). Effects of alcohol on human aggression: Validity of proposed explanations. In M. Galanter (Ed.), *Recent Developments in Alcoholism, Vol. 13: Alcohol and Violence* (pp. 227-243). New York: Plenum.

Byrnes, J. P., Miller, D. C., & Schafer, W. D. (1999). Gender differences in risk taking: A meta-analysis. *Psychological Bulletin*, **125**, 367-383

Campbell, A., Muncer, S., & Bibel, D. (2001). Women and crime: An evolutionary approach. *Aggression and Violent Behavior*, **6**, 481-497.

Campbell, H. (2000). The glass phallus: Pub(lic) masculinity and drinking in rural New Zealand. *Rural Sociology*, **65**, 562-581.

Capraro, R. L. (2000). Why college men drink: Alcohol, adventure, and the paradox of masculinity. *Journal of American College Health*, **48**, 307-315.

Caraveo-Anduaga, J. J., Colmenares-Bermudez, E., & Saldivar-Hernandez, G. J. (1999). [Gender differences in alcohol consumption in Mexico City.] *Salud Publica de Mexico*, **41**, 177-188.

Child, I. L., Barry, H., & Bacon, M. K. (1965). A cross-cultural study of drinking: III. Sex differences. *Quarterly Journal of Studies on Alcohol*, **Supplement 3**, 49-61.

Corbin, W.R., Bernat, J.A., Calhoun, K.S., McNair, L.D., & Seals, K.L. (2001). The role of alcohol expectancies and alcohol consumption among sexually victimized and nonvictimized college women. *Journal of Interpersonal Violence*, **16**, 297-311.

Courtenay, W. H. (2000). Constructions of masculinity and their influence on men's well-being: A theory of gender and health. *Social Science and Medicine*, **50**, 1385-1401.

Covington, S. S., & Surrey, J. L. (1997). The relational model of women's psychological development: Implications for substance abuse. In R. W. Wilsnack & S. C. Wilsnack (Eds.), *Gender and Alcohol: Individual and Social Perspectives* (pp. 335-351). New Brunswick, NJ: Rutgers Center of Alcohol Studies.

Dawson, D. A. (2003). Methodological issues in measuring alcohol use. *Alcohol Research & Health*, **27**, 18-29.

Dawson, D. A., & Grant, B. F. (1998). Family history of alcoholism and gender: Their combined effects on DSM-IV alcohol dependence and major depression. *Journal of Studies on Alcohol*, **59**, 97-106.

Dawson, D. A., Grant, B. F., Stinson, F. S., & Chou, P. S. (2004). Another look at heavy episodic drinking and alcohol use disorders among college and noncollege youth. *Journal of Studies on Alcohol*, **65**, 477-488.

Degenhardt, L., Hall, W., Teesson, M,; & Lynskey, M. (1997). *Alcohol Use Disorders in Australia: Findings from the National Survey of Mental Health and Well Being*. NDARC Technical Report No. 97. National Drug and Alcohol Research Centre, New South Wales, Australia.

de Lima, M. S., Dunn, J., Novo, I. P., Tomasi, E., & Reisser, A. A. P. (2003). Gender differences in the use of alcohol and psychotropics in a Brazilian population. *Substance Use and Misuse*, **38**, 51-65.

Demmel, R., & Hagen, J. (2004). The structure of positive alcohol expectancies in alcohol dependent inpatients. *Addiction Research and Theory*, **12**, 125-140.

Denny, C. H., Serdula, M. K., Holtzman, D., Nelson, D. E. (2003). Physician advice about smoking and drinking: Are U. S. adults being informed? *American Journal of Preventive Medicine*, **24**, 71-74.

DeVille, K. A., & Kopelman, L. M. (1998). Moral and social issues regarding pregnant women who use and abuse drugs. *Obstetrics and Gynecology Clinics of North America*, **25**, 237-254.

Dolgin, J. L. (1991). The law's response to parental alcohol and "crack" abuse. *Brooklyn Law Review*, **56**, 1213-1268.

Driessen, H. (1992). Drinking on masculinity: Alcohol and gender in Andalusia. In D. Gefou-Madianou (Ed.), *Alcohol, Gender and Culture* (pp. 71-79). London: Routledge.

Eckel, C. C., & Grossman, P. J. (2002). Sex differences and statistical stereotyping in attitudes toward financial risk. *Evolution and Human Behavior*, **23**, 281-295.

Engwall, D., Hunter, R., & Steinberg, M. (2004). Gambling and other risk behaviors on university campuses. *Journal of American College Health*, **52**, 245-255.

Ezzati, M., Lopez, A., Rodgers, A., Hoorn, S.V., & Murray, C.J.L. Selected major risk factors and global and regional burden of disease. *The Lancet*, **360**, 1347-1360.

Fagrell, B., De Faire, U., Bondy, S., Criqui, M., Gaziano, M., Gronbaek, M., Jackson, R., Klatsky, A., Salonen, J., & Shaper, A. G. (1999). The effects of light to moderate drinking on cardiovascular diseases. *Journal of Internal Medicine*, **246**, 331-340.

Fals-Stewart, W. (2003). The occurrence of partner physical aggression on days of alcohol consumption: A longitudinal diary study. *Journal of Consulting and Clinical Psychology*, **71**, 41-52.

Fetchenhauer, D., & Rohde, P. A. (2002). Evolutionary personality psychology and victimology: Sex differences in risk attitudes and short term orientation and their relation to sex differences in victimizations. *Evolution and Human Behavior*, **23**, 233-244.

Frezza, M., Di Padova, C., Pozzato, G., Terpin, M., Baraona, E., & Lieber, C. S. (1990). High blood alcohol levels in women: The role of decreased gastric alcohol dehydrogenase activity and first-pass metabolism. *New England Journal of Medicine*, **322**, 95-99.

Frone, M. R. (1999). Work stress and alcohol use. *Alcohol Research & Health*, **23**, 284-291.

Gefou-Madianou, D. (Ed.) (1992). *Alcohol, Gender and Culture*. New York: Routledge.

Giancola, P. R. (2002). Alcohol related aggression during the college years: Theories, risk factors and policy implications. *Journal of Studies on Alcohol*, **Supplement 14**, 129-139.

Giancola, P. R. (2003). The moderating effects of dispositional empathy on alcohol related aggression in men and women. *Journal of Abnormal Psychology*, **112**, 275-281.

Gmel, G., Bloomfield, K., Ahlström, S., Choquet, M., & Lecomte, T. (2000). Women's roles and women's drinking: A comparative study in four European countries. *Substance Abuse*, **21**, 249-264.

Gmel, G., Rehm, J., & Kuntsche, E. (2003). Binge-trinken in Europa: Epidemiologie und folgen. *Zeitschrift zur Wissenschaft und Praxis*, **49**, 105-116.

Graham, K., Plant, M., & Plant, M. (2004). Alcohol, gender and partner aggression: A general population study of British adults. *Addiction Research and Theory*, **12**, 373-384.

Graham, K., & Wells, S. (2003). "Somebody's gonna get their head kicked in tonight!": Aggression among young males in bars --- a question of values? *British Journal of Criminology*, **43**, 546-566.

Graham, K., West, P., & Wells, S. (2000). Evaluating theories of alcohol-related aggression using observations of young adults in bars. *Addiction*, **95**, 847-863.

Graham, K., Wilsnack, R. W., Dawson, D., & Vogeltanz, N. D. (1998). Should alcohol consumption measures be adjusted for gender differences? *Addiction*, **93**, 1137-1147.

Grant, B. F., Dawson, D. A., Stinson, F. S., Chou, S. P., Dufour, M. C., & Pickering, R. P. (2004). The 12-month prevalence and trends in DSM-IV alcohol abuse and dependence: United States,1991-1992 and 2001-2002. *Drug and Alcohol Dependence*, **74**, 223-234.

Grzywacz, J. G., & Marks, N. F. (2000). Family, work, work family spillover, and problem drinking during midlife. *Journal of Marriage and the Family*, **62**, 336-348.

Hajema, K.-J., & Knibbe, R. A. (1998). Changes in social roles as predictors of changes in drinking behaviour. *Addiction*, **93**, 1717-1727.

Hammill, J. (2001). The culture of masculinity in an Australian indigenous community. *Development*, **44**, 21-24.

Hansagi, H., Romelsjö, A., de Verdier, M. G., Andréasson, S., & Leifman, A. (1995). Alcohol consumption and stroke mortality: 20-year follow-up of 15,077 men and women. *Stroke*, **26**, 1768-1773.

Hao, W., Su, Z. H., Lui, B. L., Zhang, K., Yang, H. Q., Chen, S. Z., Biao, M. Z., & Cui, C. (2004). Drinking and drinking patterns and health status in the general population of five areas of China. *Alcohol and Alcoholism*, **39**, 43-52.

Harford, T. C., Wechsler, H., & Muthén, B. O. (2003). Alcohol-related aggression and drinking at off-campus parties and bars: A national study of current drinkers in college. *Journal of Studies on Alcohol*, **64**, 704-711.

Hartog, J., Ferrer-Carbonell, A., & Jonker, N. (2002). Linking measured risk aversion to individual characteristics. *Kyklos*, **55**, 3-26.

Hasin, D. S., & Grant, B. F. (2004). The co-occurrence of DSM-IV alcohol abuse in DSM-IV alcohol dependence: Results of the National Epidemiologic Survey on Alcohol and Related Conditions on heterogeneity that differ by population subgroup. *Archives of General Psychiatry*, **61**, 891-896.

Heath, A. C., Bucholz, K. K., Madden, P. A. F., Dinwiddie, S. H., Slutske, W. S., Bierut, L. J., Statham, D. J., Dunne, M. P., Whitfield, J. B., & Martin, N. G. (1997). Genetic and environmental contributions to alcohol dependence risk in a national twin sample: Consistency of findings in men and women. *Psychological Medicine*, **27**, 1381-1396.

Higuchi, S., Parrish, K. M., Dufour, M. C., Towle, L. H., & Harford, T. C. (1994). Relationship between age and drinking patterns and drinking problems among Japanese, Japanese-Americans, and Caucasians. *Alcoholism: Clinical and Experimental Research*, **18**, 305-310.

Hill, E. M., & Chow, K. (2002). Life-history theory and risky drinking. *Addiction*, **97**, 401-413.

Hirschberger, G., Florian, V., Mikulinver, M., Goldenberg, J. L., & Pyszczynski, T. (2002). Gender differences in the willingness to engage in risky behavior: A terror management perspective. *Death Studies*, **26**, 117-141.

Hunt, G. P., & Laidler, K. J. (2001). Alcohol and violence in the lives of gang members. *Alcohol Research & Health*, **25**, 66-71.

Janghorbani, M., Ho, S. Y., Lam, T. H., & Janus, E. D. (2003). Prevalence and correlates of alcohol use: A population-based study in Hong Kong. *Addiction*, **98**, 215-224.

Jhingan, H. P., Shyangwa, P., Sharma, A., Prasad, K. M. R., & Khandelwal, S. K. (2003). Prevalence of alcohol dependence in a town in Nepal as assessed by the CAGE questionnaire. *Addiction*, **98**, 339-343.

Joffe, A. H. (1998). Alcohol and social complexity in ancient western Asia. *Current Anthropology*, **39**, 297-322.

Kawakami, N., Shimizu, H., Haratani, T., Iwata, N., & Kitamura, T. (2004). Lifetime and 6 month prevalence of DSM III R psychiatric disorders in an urban community in Japan. *Psychiatry Research*, **121**, 293-301.

Kebede, D., & Alem, A. (1999). The epidemiology of alcohol dependence and problem drinking in Addis Ababa, Ethiopia. *Acta Psychiatrica Scandinavica*, **100** (Supplement 397), 30-34.

Kilpatrick, D. G., Acierno, R., Resnick, H. S., Saunders, B. E., & Best, C. L. (1997). A two-year longitudinal analysis of the relationships between violent assault and substance use in women. *Journal of Consulting and Clinical Psychology*, **65**, 834-847.

Koopman, C., Wanat, S. F., Whitsell, S., Westrup, D., & Matano, R. A. (2003). Relationships of alcohol use, stress, avoidance coping, and other factors with mental health in a highly educated workforce. *American Journal of Health Promotion*, **17**, 259-268.

Kringlen, E., Torgersen, S., & Cramer, V. (2001). A Norwegian psychiatric epidemiological study. *American Journal of Psychiatry*, **158**, 1091-1098.

Kubicka, L., Csemy, L., & Kozeny, J. (1995). Prague women's drinking before and after the "velvet revolution" of 1989: A longitudinal study. *Addiction*, **90**, 1471-1478.

Kuo, M., Adlaf, E. M., Lee, H., Gliksman, L., Demers, A., & Wechsler, H. (2002). More Canadian students drink but American students drink more: Comparing college alcohol use in two countries. *Addiction*, **97**, 1583-1592.

LaGrange, T. C., & Silverman, R. A. (1999). Low self-control and opportunity: Testing the general theory of crime as an explanation for gender differences in delinquency. *Criminology*, **37**, 41-72.

Lahelma, E., Kangas, R., & Manderbacka, K. (1995). Drinking and unemployment: Contrasting patterns among men and women. *Drug and Alcohol Dependence*, **37**, 71-82.

Laitinen, J., Ek, E., & Sovio, U. (2002). Stress-related eating and drinking behavior and body mass index and predictors of this behavior. *Preventive Medicine*, **34**, 29-39.

Leigh, B. C. (1995). A thing so fallen and so vile: Images of drinking and sexuality in women. Contemporary *Drug Problems*, **22**, 415-434.

Lundahl, L. H., Davis, T. M., Adesso, V. J., & Lukas, S. E. (1997). Alcohol expectancies: Effects of gender, age, and family history of alcoholism. *Addictive Behaviors*, **22**, 115-125.

MacLatchy-Gaudet, H. A., & Stewart, S. H. (2001). The context specific positive alcohol outcome expectancies of university women. *Addictive Behaviors*, **26**, 31-49.

MacDonald, S. (1994). Whisky, women, and the Scottish drink problem: A view from the Highlands. In M. McDonald (Ed.), *Gender, Drink and Drugs* (pp. 125-143). Providence, RI: Berg.

MacQueen, K. M., Nopkesorn, T., Sweat, M. D., Sawaengdee, Y., Mastro, T. D., & Weniger, B. G. (1996). Alcohol consumption, brothel attendance, and condom use: Normative expectations among Thai military conscripts. *Medical Anthropology Quarterly*, **10**, 402-423.

Magazine, R. (2004). Both husbands and banda (gang) members: Conceptualizing marital conflict and instability among young rural migrants in Mexico City. *Men and Masculinities*, **7**, 144-165.

Mäkelä, K., & Mustonen, H. (2000). Relationships of drinking behavior, gender, and age with reported negative and positive experiences related to drinking. *Addiction*, **95**, 727-736.

Mäkelä, P., Fonager, K., Hibbell, B., Nordlund, S., Sabroe, S., & Simpura, J. (2001). Episodic heavy drinking in four Nordic countries: A comparative survey. *Addiction*, **96**, 1575-1588.

Malet, L., Llorca, P.-M., Boussiron, D., Schwan, R., Facy, F., & Reynaud, M. (2003). General practitioners and alcohol use disorders: Quantity without quality. *Alcoholism: Clinical and Experimental Research*, **27**, 61-66.

Malyutina, S., Bobak, M., Kurilovitch, S., Nikitin, Y., & Marmot, M. (2004). Trends in alcohol intake by education and marital status in an urban population in Russia between the mid 1980s and the mid 1990s. *Alcohol and Alcoholism*, **39**, 64-69.

Malyutina, S., Bobak, M., Kurilovitch, S., Ryizova, E., Nikitin, Y., & Marmot, M. (2001). Alcohol consumption and binge drinking in Novosibirsk, Russia, 1985-1995. *Addiction*, **96**, 987-995.

Martin, A. L. (2001). *Alcohol, Sex, and Gender in Late Medieval and Early Modern Europe*. New York: Palgrave.

McClelland, D. C., Davis, W. N., Kalin, R., & Wanner, E. (1972). *The Drinking Man: Alcohol and Human Motivation*. New York: Free Press.

McKee, M., Pomerleau, J., Robertson, A., Pudule, I., Grinberga, D., Kadziauskiene, K., Abaravicius, A., & Vaask, S. (2000). Alcohol consumption in the Baltic Republics. *Journal of Epidemiology and Community Health*, **54**, 361-366.

McKee, S. A., Hinson, R. E., Wall, A.-M., & Spriel, P. (1998). Alcohol outcome expectancies and coping styles as predictors of alcohol use in young adults. *Addictive Behaviors*, **23**, 17-22.

McLaughlin, P. M. (1991). Inebriate reformatories in Scotland: An institutional history. In S. Barrows & R. Room (Eds.), *Drinking: Behavior and Belief in Modern History* (pp. 287-314). Berkeley: University of California Press.

McPherson, M., Casswell, S., & Pledger, M. (2004). Gender convergence in alcohol consumption and related problems: Issues and outcomes from comparisons of New Zealand survey data. *Addiction*, **99**, 738-748.

Mendoza-Sassi, R. A., & Beria, J. U. (2003). Prevalence of alcohol-use disorders and associated factors: A population-based study using AUDIT in southern Brazil. *Addiction*, **98**, 799-804.

Mercer, P. W., & Khavari, K. A. (1990). Are women drinking more like men? An empirical examination of the convergence hypothesis. *Alcoholism: Clinical and Experimental Research*, **14**, 461-466.

Meyer, C., Rumpf, H. J., Hapke, U., Dilling, H., & John, U. (2000). Prevalence of alcohol consumption, abuse and dependence in a country with high per capita consumption: Findings from the German TACOS study. Social Psychiatry and Psychiatric *Epidemiology*, **35**, 539-547.

Miller, J. W., Gfroerer, J. C., Brewer, R. D., Naimi, T. S., Mokdad, A., & Giles, W. H. (2004). Prevalence of adult binge drinking: A comparison of two national surveys. *American Journal of Preventive Medicine*, **27**, 197 204.

Mirand, A. L., & Welte, J. W. (1994). Total body water adjustment of mean alcohol intakes. Journal of Substance *Abuse*, **6**, 419-425.

Mohan, D., Chopra, A., & Sethi, H. (2002). Incidence estimates of substance use disorders in a cohort from Delhi, India. *Indian Journal of Medical Research*, **115**, 128-135.

Morales-Garcia, J. I. D. L. C., Fernandez- Garate, I. H., Tudon-Garces, H., la Pena, J. E. D., Zarate-Aguilar, A., & Madrazo-Navarro, M. (2002). [The prevalence of hazardous and harmful use of alcohol among the insured population of Instituto Mexicano del Seguro Social.] *Salud Publica de Mexico*, **44**, 113-121.

Morr, M. C., & Mongeau, P. A. (2004). First date expectations The impact of sex of initiator, alcohol consumption, and relationship type. *Communication Research*, **31**, 3-35.

Murdock, C. G. (2001). *Domesticating Drink: Women, Men, and Alcohol in America*, 1870 1940. Baltimore, MD: Johns Hopkins University Press.

Nayak, A. (2003). Last of the "Real Geordies"? White masculinities and the subcultural response to deindustrialisation. *Environment and Planning D: Society and Space*, **21**, 7-25.

Neff, J. A., Prihoda, T. J., & Hoppe, S. K. (1991). "Machismo," self-esteem, education, and high maximum drinking among Anglo, black, and Mexican-American male drinkers. *Journal of Studies on Alcohol*, **52**, 458-463.

Neumark, Y. D., Rahav, G., & Jaffe, D. H. (2003). Socio economic status and binge drinking in Israel. *Drug and Alcohol Dependence*, **69**, 15-21.

Neve, R. J. M., Drop, M. J., Lemmens, P. H., & Swinkels, H. (1996). Gender differences in drinking behaviour in the Netherlands: Convergence or stability? *Addiction*, **91**, 357-373.

Nghe, L. T., Mahalik, J. R., & Lowe, S. M. (2003). Influences on Vietnamese men: Examining traditional gender roles, the refugee experience, acculturation, and racism in the United States. *Journal of Multicultural Counseling and Development*, **31**, 245-261.

Nicolaides, B. M. (1996). The state's "sharp line between the sexes": Women, alcohol and the law in the United States, 1850-1980. *Addiction*, **91**, 1211-1229.

Nishimoto, R. H., & Roberts, A. C. (2001). Coercion and drug treatment for postpartum women. *American Journal of Drug and Alcohol Abuse*, **27**, 161-181.

O'Brien, S., Sinclair, H., Soni, S., O'Dowd, T., & Thomas, D. (2001). Trends in alcohol consumption in undergraduate third level students: 1992-1999. *Irish Journal of Medical Science*, **170**, 224-227.

O'Leary, K. D., & Schumacher, J. A. (2003). The association between alcohol use and intimate partner violence: Linear effect, threshold effect, or both? *Addictive Behaviors*, **28**, 1575-1585.

Osler, M., Jorgensen, T., Davidsen, M., Gronbaek, M., Bronnum-Hansen, H., Madsen, M., Gerdes, U., & Schroll, M. (2001). Socioeconomic status and trends in alcohol drinking in the Danish MONICA population, 1982-1992. *Scandinavian Journal of Public Health*, **29**, 40-43.

Parker, D. A., & Harford, T. C. (1992). Gender-role attitudes, job competition and alcohol consumption among women and men. *Alcoholism: Clinical and Experimental Research*, **16**, 159-165.

Parrott, D. J., & Giancola, P. R. (2004). A further examination of the relation between trait anger and alcohol-related aggression: The role of anger control. *Alcoholism: Clinical and Experimental Research*, **28**, 855-864.

Peltzer, K. (2002). Health behaviour among black and white South Africans. *Journal of the Royal Society for the Promotion of Health*, **122**, 187-193.

Perdrix, J., Bovet, P., Larue, D., Yersin, B., Burnand, B., & Paccaud, F. (1999). Patterns of alcohol consumption in the Seychelles Islands (Indian Ocean). *Alcohol and Alcoholism*, **34**, 773-785.

Plant, M. (1997). Alcohol throughout the ages. In M. Plant, *Women and Alcohol: Contemporary and Historical Perspectives* (pp. 32-67). London: Free Association Books.

Plant, M., Thornton, C., & Plant. M. (1999, June). *The UK case for convergence.* Paper presented at the 25th Annual Symposium of the Kettil Bruun Society for Social and Epidemiological Research on Alcohol, Montreal, Canada.

Purcell, N. (1994). Women and wine in ancient Rome. In M. McDonald (Ed.), *Gender, Drink and Drugs* (pp. 191-208). Providence, RI: Berg.

Quigley, B. M., Corbett, A. B., & Tedeschi, J. T. (2002). Desired image of power, alcohol expectancies, and alcohol related aggression. *Psychology of Addictive Behaviors*, **16**, 318-324.

Ramstedt, M. (2002). Alcohol-related mortality in 15 European countries in the postwar period. *European Journal of Population*, **18**, 307-323.

Rehm, J., Greenfield, T. K., & Rogers, J. D. (2001). Average volume of alcohol consumption, patterns of drinking, and all-cause mortality: Results from the US National Alcohol Survey. *American Journal of Epidemiology*, **153**, 64-71.

Rehm, J., Room, R., Monteiro, M., Gmel, G., Graham, K., Rehn, N., Sempos, C.T., & Jernigan, D. (2003). Alcohol as a risk factor for global burden of disease. *European Addiction Research*, **9**, 157-164.

Rijken, T., Velema, J. P., & Dijkstra, R. (1998). Alcohol consumption in the rural population of Misungwi subdistrict in Mwanza Region, Tanzania. *Journal of Studies on Alcohol*, **59**, 146-151.

Rivara, F. P., Garrison, M. M., Ebel, B., McCarty, C. A., & Christakis, D. A. (2004). Mortality attributable to harmful drinking in the United States, 2000. *Journal of Studies on Alcohol*, **65**, 530-536.

Roberts, B. (2004). Drinking like a man: The paradox of excessive drinking for 17th-century Dutch youths. *Journal of Family History*, **29**, 237-252.

Romelsjo, A., & Lundberg, M. (1996). The changes in the social class distribution of moderate and high alcohol consumption and of alcohol related disabilities over time in Stockholm County and in Sweden. *Addiction*, **91**, 1307-1323.

Rosenblitt, J. C., Soler, H., Johnson, S. E., & Quadagno, D. M. (2001). Sensation-seeking and hormones in men and women: Exploring the link. *Hormones and Behavior*, **40**, 396-402.

Sandmaier, M. (1980). Bacchantic maidens and temperance daughters. In M. Sandmaier, *The Invisible Alcoholics: Women and Alcohol Abuse in America* (pp. 24-57). New York: McGraw-Hill.

San Jose, B., Lagiou, P., Chloptsios, Y., & Trichopoulou, A. (2001). Sociodemographic correlates of abstinence and excessive drinking in the Greek population. *Substance Use and Misuse*, **36**, 463-475.

Schulenberg, J., O'Malley, P. M., Bachman, J. G., & Johnston, L. D. (2000). "Spread your wings and fly": The course of well-being and substance use during the transition to young adulthood. In L. J. Crockett & R. K. Silbereisen (Eds.), *Negotiating Adolescence in Times of Social Change* (pp. 224-255). New York: Cambridge University Press.

Scott, K. D., Schafer, J., & Greenfield, T. K. (1999). The role of alcohol in physical assault perpetration and victimization. *Journal of Studies on Alcohol*, **60**, 528-536.

Seale, J. P., Seale, J. D., Alvarado, M., Vogel, R. L., & Terry, N. E. (2002). Prevalence of problem drinking in a Venezuelan Native American population. *Alcohol and Alcoholism*, **37**, 198-204.

Serdula, M. K., Brewer, R. D., Gillespie, C., Denny, C. H., & Mokdad, A. (2004). Trends in alcohol use and binge drinking, 1985-1999: Results of a multi-state survey. *American Journal of Preventive Medicine*, **26**, 294-298.

Shore, E. R. (1997). The relationship of gender balance at work, family responsibilities and workplace characteristics to drinking among male and female attorneys. *Journal of Studies on Alcohol*, **58**, 297-302.

Siegfried, N., Parry, C. D. H., Morojele, N. K., & Wason D. (2001). Profile of drinking behaviour and comparison of self-report with the CAGE questionnaire and carbohydrate-deficient transferrin in a rural Lesotho community. *Alcohol and Alcoholism*, **36**, 243-248.

Sieri, S., Agudo, A., Kesse, E., Klipstein-Grobusch, K., San-Jose, B., Welch, A. A., Krogh, V., et al . (2002). Patterns of alcohol consumption in 10 European countries participating in the European Prospective Investigation into Cancer and Nutrition (EPIC) project. *Public Health Nutrition*, **5** (6B) (Special Issue), 1287-1296.

Singleton, N., Bumpstead, R., O'Brien, M., Lee, A., & Meltzer, H. (2003). Psychiatric morbidity among adults living in private households. *International Review of Psychiatry*, **15**, 65-73.

Skaff, M. M., Finney, J. W., & Moos, R. H. (1999). Gender differences in problem drinking and depression: Different "vulnerabilities"? *American Journal of Community Psychology*, **27**, 25-54.

Slutske, W. S., Heath, A. C., Madden, P. A. F., Bucholz, K. K., Dinwiddie, S. H., Dunne, M. P., Statham, D. S., Whitfield, J. B., & Martin, N. G. (1995). Is alcohol flushing a protective factor for alcoholism in Caucasians? *Alcoholism: Clinical and Experimental Research*, **19**, 582-592.

Slutske, W. S., Piasecki, T. M., & Hunt-Carter, E. E. (2003). Development and initial validation of the Hangover Symptoms Scale: Prevalence and correlates of hangover symptoms in college students. *Alcoholism: Clinical and Experimental Research*, **27**, 1442-1450.

Spicer, P., Beals, J., Croy, C. D., Mitchell, C. M., Novins, D. K., Moore, L., & Manson, S. M. (2003). The prevalence of DSM III R alcohol dependence in two American Indian populations. *Alcoholism: Clinical and Experimental Research*, **27**, 1785-1797.

Spigner, C., Hawkins, W., & Loren, W. (1993). Gender differences in perception of risk associated with alcohol and drug use among college students. *Women and Health*, **20**, 87-97.

Suggs, D. N. (1996). Mosadi Tshwene: The construction of gender and the consumption of alcohol in Botswana. *American Ethnologist*, **23**, 597-610.

Suggs, D. N. (2001). "These young chaps think they are just men, too": Redistributing masculinity in Kgatleng bars. *Social Science and Medicine*, **53**, 241-250.

Svikis, D. S., & Reid-Quinones, K. (2003). Screening and prevention of alcohol and drug use disorders in women. Obstetrics and Gynecology Clinics of North America, 30, 447-468.

Taillon, P. M. (2002). "What we want is good, sober men": Masculinity, respectability, and temperance in the railroad brotherhoods, c. 1870 1910. *Journal of Social History*, **36**, 319-338, 532.

Takano, T., Nakamura, K., & Watanabe, M. (1996). Increased female drinking in accordance with post industrial urbanization in Japan. *Alcohol and Alcoholism*, **31**, 41-49.

Testa, M. (2002). The impact of men's alcohol consumption on perpetration of sexual aggression. *Clinical Psychology Review*, **22**, 1239-1263.

Testa, M., & Leonard, K. E. (2001). The impact of marital aggression on women's psychological and marital functioning in a newlywed sample. *Journal of Family Violence*, **16**, 115-130.

Testa, M., Livingston, J. A., & Leonard, K. E. (2003). Women's substance use and experiences of intimate partner violence: A longitudinal investigation among a community sample. *Addictive Behaviors*, **28**, 1649 1664.

Testa, M., Vanzile-Tamsen, C., & Livingston, J. A. (2004). The role of victim and perpetrator intoxication on sexual assault outcomes. *Journal of Studies on Alcohol*, **65**, 320-329.

Thomasson, H. R. (1995). Gender differences in alcohol metabolism: Physiological responses to ethanol. In M. Galanter (Ed.), *Recent Developments in Alcoholism, Vol. 12: Alcoholism and Women* (pp. 163-179). New York: Plenum.

Thundal, K.-L., Granbom, S., & Allebeck, P. (1999). Women's alcohol dependence and abuse: The relation to social network and leisure time. *Scandinavian Journal of Public Health*, **27**, 30-37.

Tomsen, S. (1997). A top night: Social protest, masculinity, and the culture of drinking violence. *British Journal of Criminology*, **37**, 90-103.

United Nations Development Programme (2004). *World Development Report*. New York: Oxford University Press.

Vahtera, J., Poikolainen, K., Kivimaki, M., Ala Mursula, L., & Pentti, J. (2002). Alcohol intake and sickness absence: A curvilinear relation. *American Journal of Epidemiology*, **156**, 969 976.

Wall, A. M., Hinson, R. E., & McKee, S. A. (1998). Alcohol outcome expectancies, attitudes toward drinking and the theory of planned behavior. *Journal of Studies on Alcohol*, **59**, 409-419.

Wall, A. M., McKee, S. A., & Hinson, R. E. (2000). Assessing variation in alcohol outcome expectancies across environmental context: An examination of the situational specificity hypothesis. *Psychology of Addictive Behaviors*, **14**, 367-375.

Wang, C.-H., Liu, W.T., Zhang, M. Y., Yu, E.S.H., Xia, Z. Y., Fernandez, M., Lung, C. T., Xu, C. L., & Qu, G. Y. (1992). Alcohol use, abuse, and dependency in Shanghai. In J. E. Helzer and G.J. Canino (Eds.), *Alcoholism in North America, Europe, and Asia* (pp. 264 286). New York: Oxford University Press.

Warner, J. (1997). The sanctuary of sobriety: The emergence of temperance as a feminine virtue in Tudor and Stuart England. *Addiction*, **92**, 97-111.

Watten, R. G. (1997). Gender and consumption of alcohol: The impact of body composition, sensation seeking, and coping styles. *British Journal of Health Psychology*, **2** (Part 1), 15-25.

Weber, E. U., Blais, A.-R., & Betz, N. E. (2002). A domain specific risk attitude scale: Measuring risk perceptions and risk behaviors. *Journal of Behavioral Decision Making*, **15**, 263-290.

Wells, S., & Graham, K. (2003). Aggression involving alcohol: Relationship to drinking patterns and social context. *Addiction*, **98**, 33-42.

Welty, T. K., Lee, E. T., Yeh, J., Cowan, L. D., Go, O., Fabsitz, R. R., Le, N.-A., Oopik, A. J., Robbins, D. C., & Howard, B. V. (1995). Cardiovascular disease risk factors among American Indians. *American Journal of Epidemiology*, **142**, 269-287.

West, M. O. (1997). Liquor and libido: "Joint drinking" and the politics of sexual control in colonial Zimbabwe, 1920s 1950s. *Journal of Social History*, **30**, 645-667.

White, H. R., & Chen, P.-H. (2002). Problem drinking and intimate partner violence. *Journal of Studies on Alcohol*, **63**, 205-214.

Williams, P. (1998). *Progress of the National Drug Strategy: Key National Indicators: Evaluation of the National Drug Strategy, Statistical Supplement*. Canberra, Australia: Commonwealth of Australia.

Williams, R. J., & Ricciardelli, L. A. (1996). Expectancies relate to symptoms of alcohol dependence in young adults. *Addiction*, **91**, 1031-1039.

Willis, J. (1999). Enkurma sikitoi: Commoditization, drink, and power among the Maasai. *International Journal of African Historical Studies*, **32**, 339 357.

Willis, J. (2001). "Beer used to belong to older men": Drink and authority among the Nyakyusa of Tanzania. *Africa*, **71**, 373-390.

Wilsnack, R. W., & Cheloha, R. (1987). Women's roles and problem drinking across the lifespan. *Social Problems*, **34**, 231-248.

Wilsnack, R. W., Vogeltanz, N. D., Wilsnack, S. C., Harris, T. R., et al. (2000). Gender differences in alcohol consumption and adverse drinking consequences: Cross-cultural patterns. *Addiction*, **95**, 251-265.

Wilsnack, R. W., & Wilsnack, S. C. (Eds.) (1997). *Gender and Alcohol: Individual and Social Perspectives*. New Brunswick, NJ: Rutgers Center of Alcohol Studies.

Wilsnack, R. W., & Wilsnack, S. C. (1992). Women, work, and alcohol: Failures of simple theories. *Alcoholism: Clinical and Experimental Research*, **16**, 172-179.

Wilsnack, S. C., Plaud, J. J., Wilsnack, R. W., & Klassen, A. D. (1997). Sexuality, gender, and alcohol use. In R. W. Wilsnack & S. C. Wilsnack (Eds.), *Gender and Alcohol: Individual and Social Perspectives* (pp. 250-288). New Brunswick, NJ: Rutgers Center of Alcohol Studies.

Windle, M. (2003). Alcohol use among adolescents and young adults. *Alcohol Research & Health*, **27**, 79-85.

World Health Organization (2004a). *Global status report on alcohol*. Geneva: WHO.

World Health Organization (2002). *The world health report 2002*. Geneva: WHO.

World Health Organization (2004b). *The world health report 2004*. Geneva: WHO.

Yamamoto, J., Silva, J. A., Sasao, T., Wang, C., & Nguyen, L. (1993). Alcoholism in Peru. *American Journal of Psychiatry*, **150**, 1059-1062.

Yoon, Y.-H., Stinson, F. S., Yi, H-Y., & Dufour, M. C. (2003). Accidental alcohol poisoning mortality in the United States, 1996-1998. *Alcohol Research & Health*, **27**, 110-118.

York, J., & Welte, J. W. (1994). Gender comparisons of alcohol consumption in alcoholic and nonalcoholic populations. *Journal of Studies on Alcohol*, **55**, 743-750.

Zaleskiewicz, T. (2001). Beyond risk seeking and risk aversion: Personality and the dual nature of economic risk taking. *European Journal of Personality*, **15**, S105-S122.

Zhang, J., Wang, J., Lu, Y., Qiu, X., & Fang, Y. (2004). Alcohol abuse in a metropolitan city in China: A study of the prevalence and risk factors. *Addiction*, **99**, 1103-1110.

Zuckerman, M., & Kuhlman, D. M. (2000). Personality and risk-taking: Common biosocial factors. *Journal of Personality*, **68**, 999-1029.

CHAPTER 2

SOCIAL CONSEQUENCES OF
ALCOHOL CONSUMPTION IN ARGENTINA

MYRIAM I. MUNNÉ

INTRODUCTION

The Republic of Argentina is located in the southern part of South America. Its length is 3,800 km and the population is 38 million. Almost half of the population live in the Capital and Province of Buenos Aires. Ninety six percent of the population is white and principally descendants of Italian and Spanish immigrants. The literacy rate is 96.2% and the life expectancy is 70.4 years for men and 76.6 years for women.

Argentina has been facing an acute economic crisis in the last ten years. Rates of poverty and unemployment have increased dramatically. After the devaluation of the currency in December 2001, the political and social climate started to worsen. The feeling of social vulnerability was very high and the financial situation was critical. In addition, crime rates rose and the population was very concerned about security.

Alcohol related problems have been a subject of increasing awareness in Argentina in recent years. Although little research has been done, there has been public concern about alcohol related harm lately. Local norms are being redefined in order to restrict the availability of alcohol. In 2002, Argentina participated in the collaborative international project "Gender, Alcohol, and Culture: An International Study (GENACIS). The possibility of doing a survey in the general population was challenging. Despite the adverse circumstances, the survey was carried out successfully.

The aim of the present article is to analyse the social consequences of drinking. Age, gender and drinking patterns will be analysed in relation to alcohol problems. These findings will be explored taking into account the current economic crisis. Social consequences were chosen because the GENACIS survey provided the first comprehensive national data concerning different aspects of social harm related to alcohol. Firstly, an overview of alcohol consumption and alcohol problems is given, followed by the major findings of GENACIS.

ALCOHOL CONSUMPTION IN ARGENTINA

The main alcoholic beverages in Argentina are wine, beer and spirits, with the usual strengths of 5% for beer, between 12 and 13% for wine and

40% for spirits. Considering the population of 15-55 year-olds, in 1980 per capita consumption in whole litres of ethanol for spirits was 1.62, for wine 16.27 and for beer 0.77; and in 1994, per capita consumption for spirits was 0.63, for wine 10.72 and 2.10 for beer (Verruno, 1995).

In 1999 per capita consumption in whole litres for spirits was 0.42, 6.92 for wine and 2.26 for beer (WHOSIS, 2004). An examination of the situation at the beginning of 1980 shows Argentina to be among countries with the highest per capita production of wine, in the middle bracket regarding spirits and with a very low production of beer. The most important change has to do with a reorientation of consumption to different types of alcoholic beverages. While consumption of spirits and wine have decreased, consumption of beer has increased considerably in the same period. In the last two decades, wine consumption in Argentina dropped by more than half (Tendencias Económicas, 2002).

Historically, the wine industry was a family business, but in the last few years the cyclical crisis affecting the sector and the foreign capital inflow – estimated at more than US$300 million – accelerated the process of change, with foreign partners and/or owners moving into the industry. Over the last few years, producers had more chances to step up foreign sales. Local and foreign producers made important investments aimed at reconverting their vineyards to improve the quality and size of their plantations.

The beer consumed in Argentina comes from four large companies. At present, the installed capacity exceeds 26 million hectolitres/year, almost twice as much as 10 years ago. Over the last 6 years, the sector's investments have exceeded US$750 million, with the introduction of state-of-the-art technology, expansion and construction of new plants, thus increasing production and quality. The sector's leading companies have made substantial publicity investments to step up consumption, mainly supporting sports events and sports professionals in different fields. In some cases, they invested more than $15 million/year in campaigns, mainly targeted at young consumers, who became the fastest grown beer drinking segment of Argentinian society.

The local liquor industry is made up of 16 establishments devoted to the production of high alcohol content drinks. The sector underwent a profound restructuring in the last two decades, due to the income crunch and sizeable fiscal burden on sales of this type of beverage. Over the last few years, as a result of excise tax reduction for liquors in general and youth-oriented campaigns, the so-called white drinks (vodka, gin, tequila, among others) enjoyed an upswing.

ALCOHOL-RELATED PROBLEMS

Although alcohol use is a significant threat to world health (WHO,1999), there is a lack of reliable data in the country on alcohol-related harm in the population. According to available data, there were 277,148 deaths in the country in 2000. Among these, 733 (663 male, 110 female) were caused by mental and behavioural problems due to the use of alcohol (Ministry of Health, 2000). The population most affected was from 45 to 54 years of age. There were 710 (623 male, 87 female) deaths caused by alcoholic liver disease. According to the same source, cirrhosis and other chronic diseases were the fifth leading cause of death among people from 50 to 64 years of age.

Although rates of traffic accidents are very high, especially in the city of Buenos Aires, there are no reliable data available on the role of alcohol in these accidents. The same is true for homicide and suicide.

OVERVIEW OF RESEARCH FINDINGS

The first national study of use of psychoactive substances was carried out in 1999 (Míguez,1999). This study was a big advance because it provided a more complete picture of the situation at a national level. The study questionnaire was an adaptation of the 1997 WHO CIDI version 2.1 questionnaire. A representative sample of the country's population aged between 16-64 years old consisted of 2699 people, 48.3% male and 51.7 % female. Another representative sample of 356 cases was taken for the population of 12-15 year olds.

The prevalence of alcohol consumption in the last 30 days was 66.2% (78.8% male and 54.4% female). The average age at which people began to drink was 17 years old (16 for males and 18 for women). The average consumption of drinks by people who had reported to have drunk at least once a week within the last year was 4.2 (5.1 male, 2.5 female). The alcoholic beverage most consumed was beer, followed by wine and spirits. Alcohol abuse was considered as intake higher than 70g of absolute alcohol daily. Alcohol abuse by people reported to have drunk at least once a week within the last year was 13.2% (18.1% male and 4.7% female). The rate was much higher among males, and the age group with the highest rate was 16-24 year-olds. In addition, males were the ones who reported more problems, and especially males from the 16-24 year age group.

Nearly ten percent (9.9%; 13.4% male and 3.6% female) of the sample reported to have drunk in situations in which to do so was physically dangerous, such as driving, handling machinery, or similar situations (among those who reported having drunk at least once a week within the last year). In the population of 16-64 years old, alcohol abuse in the last 30 days was 6.61%, with young people in a situation of social vulnerability (low socio-economic level and education) being the ones who abused more. It must be emphasized that the rate of abuse was 7 times higher in men than in women. Alcohol dependence in people who reported having drunk in the last year was 4.3% and the patterns were similar to those for alcohol abuse (mainly males and young people in a socially vulnerable situation).

The second national study was carried out in 2004. Data is still being processed but one of the major findings is that among adolescents from 12-15 years old, lifetime prevalence of the use of alcohol was 40% among females and 38% among males. (SEDRONAR, 2004). Various partial studies demonstrated that alcohol abuse has increased among young people. A study carried out in the province of Buenos Aires showed that prevalence of alcohol abuse in the last 30 days was 29% (45% male and 12% female) among young people aged 16-29 years old (SADA, 2004).

In a study in four hospitals in the province of Buenos Aires (Míguez,1994), 7% of the consultations in the Hospital Emergency Facility were related to alcohol and other drugs; of these, 70.4 % were associated with alcoholic beverages (75% males and 54.2% females), followed by cocaine 7.4% (8.3% in males and 4.2% females), and psychopharmacological products 3.7% (1.2% males and 12.4% females). The questionnaire included a question regarding the consumption of alcohol in the previous six hours for all the people who attended the Hospital Emergency Facility. The answers were converted to absolute alcohol and 40cc was defined as a risky intake. The prevalence of those having taken in excess of this figure was 5.4%.

Another study was carried out during 1994 in hospitals across the whole country with both in-patients and patients who had been released within 30 days prior to the study (Sedronar,1994). The main cause of hospitalization in the sample studied (260 people) was associated with the consumption of alcohol and other drugs (42.3%), most often directly or indirectly related to the consumption of alcohol. The age groups which had the highest consumption were from 35-44 years old and 45-54 years old (25% each).

SOCIAL PERCEPTION OF ALCOHOL PROBLEMS AMONG THE GENERAL POPULATION

A study of the perception of families from Buenos Aires about drugs (Necchi, 1990) revealed that illegal drugs were condemned much more than the legal, socially accepted drugs. The occasional use of illegal substances such as cocaine or marijuana was considered much more dangerous than the use of alcoholic beverages. It seemed that what was regarded as more dangerous was the social transgression and not so much the toxicity of the substance.

A survey carried out in a sample of 7200 people above 14 years old from the whole country (APNA,1994) examined the social perception of alcohol and drug problems. Many aspects of alcohol and drug related problems were explored. A majority (82.3%) of those interviewed considered that alcohol and drug related problems have worsened in the last few years. The majority of them thought that the problems associated with alcohol and drug consumption were due to problems within the family. Regarding the official approach, 72.4% thought that there was a lack of state policies.

This perception of the problem is consistent with a survey carried out among professionals dealing with alcohol and drug problems (Munné,1996). The majority of the interviewees mentioned "health policies" as the most important health issue in Argentina. This would imply that health is not limited to disease but rather it refers to the pursuit of general well-being, and therefore that an appropriate policy is needed. Some of the interviewees stated that public policies do not exist, others pointed out the lack of organization and programmes. The lack of human and material resources was also mentioned, as well as low credibility in the role the state plays in alcohol and drug-related problems. The role of education and the mass media has also been criticized and the majority believed that the two are limited to informing in a partial way and at times to disinforming. However, they recognized the greater role education and mass-media could play if only they were better oriented towards the integral promotion of health. Alcohol and tobacco advertising was seen to be another element contributing to the increase of consumption, and the majority of the interviewees felt that tighter regulations in this regard were necessary.

LEGISLATION IN ARGENTINA

Since 1997, the country has had the "National Law of the fight against alcoholism" (n°24.788), which after years of debate, was introduced on 31 March 1997. This law states that a) it is forbidden countrywide to sell any kind of alcoholic beverage to people under the age of 18; b) it is in the national interest to fight against the excessive use of alcohol; c) it is forbidden to consume alcoholic beverages in the streets, stadiums or other places where sporting, education or cultural activities are being held; d) commercial alcoholic beverages produced in the country must have the alcoholic strength printed on the label of the container and also must say "Drink with moderation" and "Forbidden to be sold to minors under 18."

There are also restrictions placed on the advertising of alcoholic beverages, in that: a) it should not be aimed at minors under 18, b) minors under 18 should not be portrayed drinking, c) the consumption of alcohol should not suggest the improvement of physical or intellectual performance and d) alcohol should not be connected with sexual stimulation or violence in any form. This law also created the National Program for Prevention and Fight Against the Excessive Consumption of Alcohol. The Federal Council of Education and Culture is in charge of the educational aspects of the programme. Issues related to the excessive consumption of alcohol must be incorporated into all levels of education.

Public and Private institutions must have primary prevention and early detection programmes related to the pathology of the excessive consumption of alcohol. Social security services must deal with psychological, pharmacological and medical treatments related to the disease of the excessive consumption of alcohol. They must offer assistance and rehabilitation to alcoholic patients and must have prevention programmes. This law also prohibits driving any type of motor vehicle with a blood alcohol level greater than 500mg per litre of blood. In the case of a motorbike, it is prohibited to drive with a blood alcohol level greater than 200 mg per litre of blood. Public transport and commercial cargo drivers are prohibited from having any traces of alcohol in their blood stream.

Although there has not been any study on the impact of the law, there is strong evidence that the enforcement of the law is very poor. In terms of alcohol availability to minors, a study demonstrated that they can easily access alcoholic drinks in discos and other outlets (Munné, 2001a). Many cardboard boxes (one packaging in which wine is delivered) don't have any label printed indicating the alcoholic strength nor the prohibition to sell it to minors.

Social control regarding the state of being drunk in public has changed in the last year. Argentina had until last year police edicts regarding drunkenness. Policemen had the authority to detain a drunken person in the streets. If that individual showed signs of chronic alcohol dependence, the police doctor could order his confinement in a psychiatric clinic. Since March 1999, the edicts were annulled and the city of Buenos Aires now has a "Code of mutual coexistence". This code regulates minor infractions. Being drunk is not an infraction in itself any more, but if a person who has committed an infraction is intoxicated with alcohol or other substances the competent authority must bring the person immediately to an assistance centre.

Argentinian legislation does not contemplate the use of alcohol as either aggravating or attenuating responsibility for crimes. The recurrent standard is that of "imputability", which is determined by psychiatric examination of the subject. The current tendency (except in the cases of alcohol dependent people) resultant from psychiatric examinations indicates that the influence of alcohol while having committed a crime does not bear any weight to the subject´s imputability.

ALCOHOL POLICIES

In Argentina, although several national agencies are dealing with the prevention and treatment of alcohol problems, very little funds are given compared to what is assigned for illicit drugs. In addition, the prevalent policy has been assigning funds for treatment (especially for illicit drugs) and resources allocated for research have been practically nonexistent.

Prevention campaigns have been fragmented. Controls especially for drinking-driving have been implemented temporarily, especially in summer time when there is a big influx of cars on the Argentinian roads. In relation to treatment, very few hospitals have treatment units for alcohol problems. AA groups are established and are spread through the whole country. They gather usually in churches.

Regulations on taxes have changed with different governments. As happens in other developing countries such as Mexico (Riley and Marshall, 1999), there are opposite interests not only between the health authorities and the alcohol industry, but also among different sectors of government. There is a lack of an adequate national policy. A comprehensive national programme should articulate actions that could be put in practice in different areas such as health, education, social services, etc.

GENDER ROLES IN THE ARGENTINIAN SOCIETY

Although relationships between men and women have changed in the past decades, in Argentina as in other developing countries (Room et al, 2002) traditional male attitudes or "machismo" still exist. Traditionally, the man was the one who had to provide all or almost all of the total household income.

Partly due to the economic crisis, this situation has started to change, consequently gender roles are being redefined. Drinking was traditionally a male issue with women controlling men's drinking. This situation today is that , especially among the young generation, the gender gap in drinking is decreasing.

THE GENACIS STUDY

Gender, Alcohol and Culture: An International Study (GENACIS) is a collaborative multinational study designed by the International Research Group on Gender and Alcohol (IRGGA). The research instrument consists of a questionnaire divided into the following sections: demographics, work experiences, social networks, drinking variables, familial and other drinking contexts, drinking consequences, intimate relations and sexuality, violence/victimization and health and lifestyle.

The aims of GENACIS are among others:

- to compare drinking patterns between men and women
- to compare the prevalence of alcohol-related problems between men and women
- to assess the level of heavy drinking among men and women

In Argentina the original questionnaire was used with few changes. Drinking in the street was added in the section on contexts of drinking and in the question on "how much drinking is o.k" in different situations. Some questions were included in order to find out the opinions of the general population in relation to alcohol and the economic crisis (Munné, 2003). There were the following statements and people had to answer if they strongly agree, somewhat agree, somewhat disagree or strongly disagree:

In the crisis situation:

(a) the people I know drink more as a way of escaping from their problems;

(b) it is important to cut down on drinking and other expenses that are not necessary;

(c) the people I know have stopped going to bars and restaurants and now they drink at home or at a friend's home;

(d) the people I know buy cheaper alcoholic drinks and/or of less quality.

METHOD

SAMPLE

The sample was selected from the city of Buenos Aires and the Province of Buenos Aires, a region that constitutes around 50% of the population of the whole country. The sample size was 1000 with a response rate of 73.65 %. The population sampled was urban males and females aged between 18 and 65 years old. Sampling involved several stages: sampling of areas and buildings, sampling of households when there were more than one household in the same building and sampling of an individual in the household.

PROCEDURE

Data collection was through face to face interviews. The questionnaire was piloted with a sample of 30. Only a few changes were made to the final version of the questionnaire before starting the fieldwork. Previous experience in surveys was one of the main considerations in the selection of interviewers. The interviewers were psychologists, anthropologists, sociologists and social workers, and a few were university students. Most of them were women. Apart from the training, the interviewers were given a "Manual for interviewers," a sheet with different community resources on alcohol and drugs, agencies dealing with domestic violence, a letter of presentation and their identification card. The Manual included the objectives of the study, issues concerning techniques for interviews (including privacy, confidentiality, reliability), how to take control of the interview, and how to behave with the sensitive parts of the questionnaire. Fieldwork started on September 25 and was completed by the end of November 2002.

RESULTS

SOCIO-DEMOGRAPHIC CHARACTERISTICS

Gender, age and education: Table 1 shows the general demographic characteristics of the sample by gender. The gender composition was 47.7% male and 52.3% female. Most of the males were in the 18-29 age-group, but females were more equally distributed among the three age-groups. Most participants had eight or more years of education and the whole sample consisted of white people.

Marital status: In terms of marital status, 39.5% of the respondents were married and 13.7% were living with a partner. Women were more likely to be married or living with a partner than men. Among the people who were not married or living with a partner, 32.1 % (39.1% male, 23.7% female) had at the time of the survey a close romantic relationship and 64.5% (60.2% male, 69.7% female) did not. Among those who had a close romantic relationship, 79.6% of men had a female partner and 88.7% of women had a male partner. Thus people that declared to have

TABLE 1.   General demographic characteristics by gender

Characteristics	Male (402) %	Female (598) %
Age		
18-29 years old	47.2	33.1
30-44 years old	22.4	33.5
45+ years old	30.4	33.4
Education		
None	0.5	0.1
<8 years	35.3	31.1
8+years	64.2	68.8
Marital Status		
Married/lives with partner	46.4	59.4
Divorced/separated	7.6	18.5
Not married	42.9	19.5
Widowed	3.1	2.6
Religion		
Catholic	78.3	85.5
No religious preference	17.8	9.7
Employment		
Working for pay	63.2	39.6
Involuntarily unemployed	22.1	14.2

homosexual partners were very rare (1.9% for men and 0.8% for women).

Religion: More than eighty (82.1%; 78.3% male, 85.5% female) were Catholic and 3.9% (3.2% male, 4.5% female) from other religions; 13.5% (17.8% male, 9.7% female) did not have any religious preference.

Occupation and income: Eighteen percent of the sample were involuntarily unemployed (22.1% male, 1.2% female). Due to the acute economic crisis in Argentina at the time of the study, there was each month an increasing level of unemployment and/or under unemployment. The average amount of time that people had been unemployed was 18 months. Almost half of the sample considered their work situation at least somewhat stressful. For 32.9% of the sample, household income was very low and 21.1% low. This variable was constructed according to data from INDEC (National Institute of Statistics).

Social networks: The majority of the interviewees (59%) had informal or supportive contacts with relatives, friends and others daily or almost daily and 14.8% several times a week in the 30 days prior to the survey. Only 2.9% did not have any contact at all with relatives, friends, etc.

Women reported that they felt lonely "very often" more than twice as often as men. An analysis of the data by region showed that people in the city of Buenos Aires felt much more lonely very often (20.7%) than people of Greater Buenos Aires (9.2%), and the rest of the province (6.1%).

Relatives and friends of the interviewees often lived in the same neighbourhood (50.2%) or at least in the same city (30%). The rest lived in the same region or country and only 2.1% lived in another country.

Only 20.6 % (16.3% male, 23.8% female) were members of an association or church. The figures were lower among 18 to 29 year-olds (15.7%) and people living in the city of Buenos Aires (13.8%).

DRINKING PATTERNS

Alcohol use is widespread; 84.5% of the sample were current drinkers. Table 2 shows drinking history by age and gender. Rates of abstention were: former drinker, 12.6% and lifetime abstainer, 2.9%. Women, and particularly women over 30, were the most likely to be former drinkers (30% among those 30-44, 20% among those aged 45+).

In terms of frequency of drinking, 50% of the sample drank at least once a month, and 36% at least once a week. Altogether, 30% had consumed five or more drinks at least once in the last year, and 26% reported that their usual amount per occasion was three or more drinks. Men were more likely than women to engage in each of these behaviours. Thus 56% of the men but 26% of the women drank weekly or more often, 65% of the men but 13% of the women had drunk 5+ drinks in the last year,

TABLE 2.   Drinking history by age and gender

Drinking history	Total (1000)	Male			Female		
		18-29 years old (133)	30-44 years old (139)	45+ years old (130)	18-29 years old (150)	30-44 years old (200)	45+ years old (248)
Lifetime abstainer	2.9	0.6	4.6	0.1	1.6	5.6	5.4
Former drinker	12.6	2.0	3.6	10.1	8.9	30.2	20.2
Current drinker	84.5	97.4	91.8	89.8	89.4	64.1	74.4

and 48% of the men but 11% of the women usually drank 3+ drinks.

In Table 3, the distributions of abstention and of these three drinking patterns across demographic categories are shown for men and for women. Heavier drinking is predominantly associated with youth among both men and women, particularly for women, while abstention is least common among those aged less than 30, and is most heavily associated with older age among men. Male abstainers are more likely to have less than 8 years of education, while female abstainers are predominantly

TABLE 3.   Aspects of drinking by gender and demographic characteristics

Demographics	Male				Female			
	Abstainers (34)	Weekly (224)	Usual Quantity 3+ (193)	5+ drinks (260)	Abstainers (157)	Weekly (140)	Usual quantity 3+ (65)	5+ drinks (78)
	%	%	%	%	%	%	%	%
Age								
18-29 years old	19.9	49.8	57.2	52.4	14.6	28.0	72.4	69.2
30-44 years old	29.9	20.8	24.9	26.6	49.9	28.8	15.6	18.0
45+ years old	50.2	29.4	17.9	21.0	35.5	43.2	12.0	12.8
Education								
None	0.0	0.0	1.0	0.9	0.0	0.8	0.9	0.0
<8 years	60.6	22.8	28.8	31.3	28.0	22.4	54.1	66.0
8+ years	39.4	77.1	70.2	67.8	71.9	76.7	45.0	33.7
Marital Status								
Married/lives with partner	46.5	53.2	46.6	50.3	62.8	59.4	35.8	34.2
Divorced/ Separated	27.3	3.6	4.5	5.8	24.3	6.0	41.4	46.7
Not married	26.3	41.6	48.0	42.6	8.0	32.9	22.5	19.1
Widowed	0.0	1.6	0.9	1.3	5.0	1.7	0.3	0.0
Employment								
Working for pay	82.5	62.1	60.1	57.9	42.5	49.6	22.4	26.7
Involuntarily Unemployed	9.8	23.9	25.6	24.7	5.3	8.0	38.6	45.1

better educated. Conversely, the relatively few women drinking 5+ drinks mostly have less education, while males drinking that much have more education. Frequent drinkers have better education among both men and women. Married women but not men are underrepresented among heavier drinkers, while heavier drinking women include high proportions of the divorced or separated. The unemployed are underrepresented among abstainers, while they are overrepresented particularly among heavier-drinking men.

TYPOLOGY OF DRINKING

Considering the frequency of drinking in the past 12 months and the proportions drinking 5+ drinks or not, the following typology was used. (See Table 4).

Current abstainer: Never had a drink or had none in the past year.

Infrequent light drinker: drinking less than weekly, always less than 5 drinks per occasion.

Frequent light drinker: drinking weekly + less than 5 drinks per occasion.

Infrequent heavy drinker: drinking less than weekly, sometimes 5+ drinks per occasion.

Frequent heavy drinker: drinking weekly + 5+ drinks per occasion.

As shown in Table 4, there were almost no women in the heaviest drinking group, while this pattern was more common among older than

TABLE 4. **Typology of drinking by age and gender**

	Total	Male			Female		
		18-29 years old	30-44 years old	45+ years old	18-29 years old	30-44 years old	45+ years old
	(1000)	(133)	(139)	(130)	(150)	(200)	(248)
Current abstainer	15.5	2.6	8.2	10.2	10.6	35.9	25.6
Infrequent light	43.2	27.8	21.6	38.9	57.0	48.3	55.5
Frequent light	7.5	3.2	3.1	12.4	3.3	8.3	13.6
Infrequent heavy	31.4	58.9	59.5	31.2	29.1	6.8	5.3
Frequent heavy	2.4	2.6	6.1	7.1	0.0	0.6	0.0

Note: The current abstainer category includes lifetime abstainers and former drinkers.

younger men. Over half of men under age 45 qualified as infrequent heavier drinkers, while among women there were substantial numbers in this category only among those under age 30. A majority of women were infrequent lighter drinkers, with abstention also common among those aged 30 or more. Among men aged 45 or older, about half also were either abstainers or infrequent lighter drinkers.

DRINKING CONTEXTS

The contexts in which drinking occurs are very important to analyse because they give useful information from a cultural and public health perspectives. While in some cultures people only drink on weekends and in bars (without a meal), in the Argentinian culture alcohol is integrated into daily life: 38% of men and 19.1% of women drank alcohol at a meal at least weekly. This pattern shows some differences by age groups: people from 18-29 years old drank less often at a meal than the older age groups.

For both men and women most of the drinking was done in the respondent's own home, followed by a friend's home. Drinking in bars and discos was frequent for the younger age-groups. For men, drinking in the streets was more frequent than drinking in restaurants: 3.9 % drank in the street at least weekly and mainly in the younger age-groups. It was more tolerated for males to get drunk in the street than in other situations. Public drinking, especially binge drinking increases the possibility of several drinking consequences such as interpersonal violence, accidents, etc. As drinking is a social act, the company in which people drink needs our attention, especially concerning gender roles.

Women drank more frequently with their spouses or a family member than with other people. Men drank as often with their spouse as with friends, followed by the company of a family member.

One of the greatest differences between both sexes was drinking with friends. Men tend to gather with their friends and drinking is part of this context much more frequently than for women. While 27.5% of men drank at least weekly with friends,7.3% of women did.

Again, for the Argentinian society drinking with friends in the street and eventually getting drunk was a much more common situation than drinking with friends after work before going home. The latter, a common situation in Western Europe, Canada and USA is a custom that started not long ago in the city of Buenos Aires and is practised by people in the middle and high classes. Bars featuring happy hours are widespread in downtown Buenos Aires, especially Irish pubs.

Drinking alone was much higher in men: 12.7% drank alone at least weekly while only 1.7 % of women did so. If we consider drinking with friends and alone, a considerable proportion of men's drinking is done without the potential control of a woman.

DRINKING CONSEQUENCES

There has been much research on the consequences drinking may have for people. These consequences are also mediated by cultural factors, gender roles and the beliefs and myths people may have about the effects of alcohol.

As in other studies (e.g., Wilsnack, R. et al., 2000), men reported more positive consequences of drinking as well as more negative consequences: 25.9% of men and 4.8% of women found it easier to be open with other people when they drank. Regarding sexuality, men felt less inhibited about sex while drinking as well as being more likely to feel sexually attractive than women. Almost nine percent (8.6%) of men considered it usually true that they became more aggressive towards people after drinking, while only 0.2% of women felt this way.

Partner aggression was also explored in the study. Among the people who experienced physical aggression from the partner, 12% of males and 7.2% of females had been drinking before the incident. The relationship between alcohol consumption and violence (especially domestic violence) is considered to be strong by the Argentinian culture and many times violence is justified by the consumption of alcohol (Munné,1999).

In relation to general health problems, only 9.7% of the population reported one or more health problems in the last year (34.5% for men in the 18-29 age brackets). Men reported having better physical health than women. This situation was repeated concerning mental and emotional health: women tended to report poorer mental and emotional health than men did. This may suggest that women are under more stressful situations or that they are more aware of their problem. As in many other countries, in Argentina the percentage of women seeking help in psychology clinics is much higher than men. Although 7.3% of the sample reported a harmful effect of drinking on their physical health, only 0.2% reported having an illness connected with drinking.

Questions from the CAGE questionnaire, which screens for alcohol dependence, were also explored. Altogether, 7.6% in the general population and 21.3% in the younger age group of males answered positively to two or more items in this questionnaire.

Respondents were also asked questions from the AUDIT questionnaire, and were scored on the seven last items (concerned with dependence symptoms or alcohol-related problems) as an indicator of harmful use of alcohol. In total, 11.6 % of the sample responded positively to 2 or more of these items.

Looking in depth at the AUDIT questions, the highest rate of positive response was for "not being able to stop drinking once started", which was 11.8 % in the general population. It was particularly high in the younger age group, with almost no differences between male and females (24.1% male, 20.9% female). No other consequence of drinking was reported at such a rate by men and women.

Another question in the AUDIT, "having been unable to remember what happened the night before" merits attention from the perspective of social consequences. The rate was 10.2% in the overall sample and 30.2 % in the younger group of men.

Suggestions by relatives, friends or doctor to cut down drinking were also surveyed. The figure was 9.6% for the general population and again much higher for young men (25.5%). Six percent of the sample tried to cut down their drinking but were unable to do so; the figure for young men was 15.7%. 7.3% of men and 0% of women considered seeking help for own alcohol related problems. Among those who considered seeking help, 93% received it in the past 12 months, which means that once men considered seeking help they found it, probably in the health care system or as informal help from relatives and others.

The survey explored "how much a person in different situations should feel free to drink". Men thought that getting drunk was sometimes all right much more often than women do. In fact, drunkenness was almost not tolerated at all by women. But maybe the most interesting aspect is that for women a man out at a bar with friends was the situation in which they thought most frequently that getting drunk is sometimes all right (2.3%), while for a woman out at a bar with friends the percentage was 0.3%. Although women's drinking has traditionally been condemned by Argentinian society (Munné, 2001 b), men were more tolerant of women's drunkenness with friends (5.1%).

The gap between what people consider acceptable to drink in different situations and what they actually do is a big one. One possible line of further analysis would be what drunkenness means in the Argentinian society and how many drinks would be considered the limit for a person to be considered drunk.

SOCIAL CONSEQUENCES OF ALCOHOL CONSUMPTION

A number of social consequences of alcohol consumption were also explored. The problems were grouped as follows: relationship problems, work problems, pressures to cut down, other social harms (see Tables 5 and 6). The tables show the proportions responding concerning each item that it had occurred in the last year.

As shown in Table 5, rates of relationship problems were considerable, especially for men in the age group 18-29 years old. Nearly a quarter (22.8%) of this group had problems with their marriage or their intimate relationships; 23.2% had problems with other family members. On the other hand, very few women reported having relationships problems. "People annoyed you by criticizing your drinking" was the most reported relationship problem: 26.7 % of men in the age group from 18-29 years old reported having this problem. Another important relationship problem was "spouse threatened to leave you because of your

TABLE 5. Social consequences: relationship and work by age and gender (current drinkers only)

ALCOHOL PROBLEMS	Total (809) %	Male			Female		
		18-29 years old (124) %	30-44 years old (127) %	45+ years old (117) %	18-29 years old (120) %	30-44 years old (151) %	45+ years old (170) %
RELATIONSHIPS							
Marriage/intimate relationships	**7.7**	22.8	11.8	2.6	0.0	0.0	0.0
Relationship with other family members	**8.1**	23.2	8.2	1.7	2.2	0.8	2.0
Friendships or social life	**5.7**	17.1	6.9	0.1	0.5	0.0	2.0
People annoyed you by criticizing your drinking	**9.3**	26.7	14.8	2.7	1.0	0.0	0.1
Spouse threatened to leave you because of your drinking	**6.5**	21.4	5.9	1.9	0.0	0.0	0.0
Lost a friendship	**5.2**	17.2	6.0	0.1	0.2	0.0	0.0
WORK							
Harmful effect on work, studies or employment opportunities	**5.6**	19.8	4.0	0.0	0.0	0.0	0.0
Harmful effect on housework or chores around the house	**0.6**	1.4	0.1	0.1	0.0	0.0	1.4
Lost a job or nearly lost it	**5.9**	18.5	9.2	0.0	0.0	0.0	0.0

drinking". Once again the figure was very high for the younger age group of males (21.4%).

In relation to work problems, 19.8% of men in the age group 18-29 years old reported that their drinking had harmful effect on work, studies or employment opportunities versus 4% of the group of 30-44 year-olds. Women did not report work problems, and only 1.4% reported harmful effect on housework or chores around the house in the age group of 45+ years old.

Table 6 shows that many respondents reported "pressures to cut down", especially pressures from spouse/partner; 28.4% of the younger age group of men reported having been asked to cut down by their partners. This figure was also high for females in the younger age group (22.1%).

TABLE 6. **Social consequences: pressures to cut down and other social harms by age and gender (current drinkers only)**

PRESSURES TO CUT DOWN	Total (809)	Male			Female		
		18-29 years old (124)	30-44 years old (127)	45+ years old (117)	18-29 years old (120)	30-44 years old (151)	45+years old (170)
Spouse/partner	14.2	28.4	15.9	4.0	22.1	2.7	0.0
Child	2.3	1.4	7.8	4.3	0.9	1.0	0.6
Female family member	8.8	28.2	9.4	1.3	0.9	0.1	0.0
Male family member	2.6	6.8	3.7	0.4	1.5	0.8	0.0
Someone at work or school	4.9	17.0	3.7	0.1	0.0	0.1	0.0
Female friend	4.8	17.2	0.1	0.1	1.7	0.0	0.0
Male friend	5.7	18.3	6.9	0.4	0.0	0.0	0.4
OTHER SOCIAL HARMS							
Got in a fight while drinking	8.2	23.2	9.7	1.9	2.5	0.0	2.0
Harmful effect on finances	6.2	20.0	5.5	2.2	0.1	0.0	0.1
Trouble with law about drink and driving	0.5	1.3	1.0	0.0	0.0	0.1	0.0

Women played an important role in these "pressures" — both female family members and female friends. Especially for the young men, 28.2% reported having had pressures from a female family member and 17.2% had pressures from a female friend. For the younger age group of men, a male friend also played a role in pressure to cut down (18.3%).

Concerning other social harms, men reported having been involved in a fight while drinking, especially men in the age group of 18-29 years (23.2%). Harmful effects on finances was also considerable in this group (20%).

In relation to level of education, in all of the alcohol problems analysed here, the highest figures were for people who had not finished high school. As shown in Table 7, 9.9% of current drinkers reported 3 or more alcohol problems; the highest figure was for the males in the younger age group (27.3%). Among women too, those who reported more problems were in the younger age group. In this group 26% reported at least one social consequence.

Tables 8 and 9 show that when we analysed the alcohol problems by current drinkers and 5+ drinkers, the heavier drinkers reported more

TABLE 7. Number of reported drinking-related social consequences by gender and age (current drinkers only)

Number of social consequences	Total (809) %	Male			Female		
		18-29 years old (124) %	30-44 years old (127) %	45+ years old (117) %	18-29 years old (120) %	30-44 years old (151) %	45+ years old (170) %
3 or more	9.9	27.3	14.8	2.7	1.3	0.8	2.1
2	2.0	3.2	3.5	1.3	3.0	0.0	0.0
1	8.1	8.4	3.1	5.9	21.7	2.4	2.3
0	80.0	61.1	78.5	90.1	73.9	96.9	95.6

alcohol problems than others. This was the case for almost all problems and for both male and female drinkers.

In a country under a profound economic crisis, social consequences of

TABLE 8. Relationship and work problems by current drinking and 5+ drinking

ALCOHOL PROBLEMS	Total (809) %	Male		Female	
		Current drinkers (368) %	5+drinkers (260) %	Current drinkers (441) %	5+drinkers (78) %
RELATIONSHIPS					
Marriage/intimate relationships	7.7	14.5	21.3	0.0	0.0
Relationship with other family members	8.1	13.7	19.9	1.8	9.6
Friendships or social life	5.7	9.9	17.6	0.9	3.6
People annoyed you by criticizing your drinking	9.3	17.1	25.7	0.4	1.0
Spouse threatened to leave you because of your drinking	6.5	12.3	17.6	0.0	0.0
Lost a friendship	5.2	9.7	16.4	0.1	0.3
WORK					
Harmful effect on work, studies or employment opportunities	5.6	10.6	14.7	0.0	0.0
Harmful effect on housework or chores around the house	0.6	0.7	1.3	0.4	0.0
Lost a job or nearly lost it	5.9	11.1	15.5	0.0	0.0

TABLE 9. **Pressures to cut down and other social harms by current drinking and 5+ drinking**

PRESSURES TO CUT DOWN	Total (809)	Male		Female	
		Current drinkers (368)	5+drinkers (260)	Current drinkers (441)	5+drinkers (78)
	%	%	%	%	%
Spouse/partner	14.2	18.6	27.8	9.4	47.6
Child	2.3	3.6	5.5	1.8	4.0
Female family member	8.8	16.3	24.3	0.4	1.9
Male family member	2.6	4.3	4.0	0.8	3.7
Someone at work or school	4.9	9.2	15.5	0.0	0.1
Female friend	4.8	8.5	14.3	0.7	0.9
Male friend	5.7	10.6	17.7	0.1	0.0
OTHER SOCIAL HARMS					
Got in a fight while drinking	8.2	14.0	20.3	1.6	9.0
Harmful effect on finances	6.2	11.6	16.7	0.1	0.0
Trouble with law about drink and driving	0.5	0.8	1.4	0.0	0.0

drinking would be expected to aggravate the situation. The majority of the interviewees agreed that it was important to cut down on drinking and other expenses that are not necessary (65.7% strongly agreed with this statement). To the statement on whether people bought cheaper alcoholic drinks which were of less quality, 32.4% of the sample strongly agreed and 25.9% somewhat agreed.

DISCUSSION AND CONCLUSION

Alcohol use is widespread in Argentina. The majority of the sample in this study (84.5%) were current drinkers and 50% of these drank at least once a month. As in other cultures, men drank more quantity and more frequently than women. The younger age group was the one that consumed more alcohol. Most of the drinking was done in the respondent's own home and at friend's home. Men reported more positive consequences of drinking as well as more negative consequences. AUDIT scores showed that 11.6% of the sample was considered to have a harmful use of alcohol, and 9.7% reported one or more health problems (34.5% for men in the 18-29 age bracket). Analysis of CAGE scores showed that 7.6 % of the sample could be considered to have alcohol dependence. Concerning social consequences of drinking, 9.9% of current drinkers reported 3 or more social consequences of drinking (27.3% for men aged 18-29 years).

Harmful effects of drinking on the respondent's relationships were considerable, especially in relation to marriage and intimate relationships and relationships with family members. The figures were significant among men in the younger age group. An important aspect regarding relationship problems was the issue "people annoyed you by criticizing your drinking". This figure was the highest of relationship problems.

Responses to this issue need further analysis for a better understanding of the Argentinian meaning of being annoyed by the criticisms of others towards their drinking. There are at least two possibilities: a high social control (at least from women) and the feeling of doing something bad which is connected to another question (on having a feeling of guilt or remorse after drinking) which was also high: 9.6% in the general population and higher among younger men (25.2%).

This is also related to another aspect of social consequences, the pressure to cut down, which occurred often from spouse/partner, but also from family members, especially females. The threat of the partner leaving because of drinking was also one of the major relationship problems among men. Nevertheless, it could be argued that although relatively high informal social controls exist, there is little effect on drinking, since receiving more pressure is positively associated with heavier drinking.

Problems in relation with work were nearly exclusively a male issue; 5.9% lost a job or nearly lost it because of their drinking. This figure was considerably higher for men in the younger age group (18.5%). This is a particularly harmful social consequence of drinking considering the economic situation in the country at the time of the study, where a person who lost a job was unlikely to find another one. As earlier studies have shown (e.g., Mustonen,2000) young people were more likely to report problems of all sorts related to alcohol use.

From a public health perspective, the findings of this study indicate that alcohol related problems are considerable in Argentina. More in-depth analyses are needed, especially those looking at patterns of drinking in relationship with problems of alcohol use. Qualitative analysis might contribute significantly to our understanding of drinking patterns, especially for a cross-cultural comparison.

Social harms are mediated by cultures (Partanen, 1991). Thus there is a need to explore further meanings of alcohol use and abuse in the Argentinian society. It is important to analyse alcohol problems within the culture and the historical moment that these problems occur. Lately, one of the most important changes in alcohol epidemiology has been a new recognition that patterns of drinking, as well as level of drinking are important in the links between alcohol and health (Room, 1996; 2001).

Patterns of drinking are changing and this can be seen as underlying some of the cultural differences in social definitions of alcohol problems.

Although this survey has taught us that sensitive questions such as on sexuality and violence have been answered by respondents, there is a need to explore better ways of getting the information we are trying to obtain. The responses of informants are mediated by social expectations, and thus special adaptations to local uses and norms are required when using internationally developed measures (WHO,2000). Underestimation by the respondent is more likely to occur where the behaviour in question is potentially discreditable, just as there may be overestimation where the behaviour is positively regarded (Room et al., 2002).

In conclusion, research remains the essential tool to achieve a better understanding of alcohol use and misuse and the basis to build up an adequate and successful health policy. To minimize the harm from drinking, an integrated policy is needed to articulate actions that could be put in practice in different areas such as health, education, and social services (Edwards, 1997).

ACKNOWLEDGEMENTS

The author is truly grateful to Robin Room for his suggestions and Isidore Obot for his assistance throughout the project leading to this paper. Special thanks are due to the project team in Argentina that made the survey possible.

REFERENCES

APNA (1994). Asociación de Profesionales para la nueva Argentina (Association of professionals for Argentina) *Encuesta nacional de drogadicción* (National survey of drugs) Buenos Aires: APNA.

Edwards, G , et al. (1997) *Alcohol y Salud Publica,* Spanish version of *Alcohol Policy and the Public Good.* Barcelona: J.R. Prous.

Miguez, H. (1994). El abuso de alcohol y drogas en la consulta hospitalaria de la provincia de Buenos Aires (Abuse of alcohol and drugs in hospital consultations in the province of Buenos Aires) *Revista de Salud, Prevención y Sociedad,* Año 6, **6**, 13-22.

Miguez. H. (1999). *Estudio Nacional sobre sustancias adictivas de la República Argentina.* (National Study of Adictive Substances in Argentina). Buenos Aires: SEDRONAR, Secretaría de Programación para la Prevención de la Drogadicción y Lucha contra el Narcotráfico (National Secretary for the Prevention of Drug-addiction and Fight against Drug trafficking).

Ministry of Health (2000). *Estadísticas Vitales. Información Básica* (Basic Statistical Information) Nº44. Buenos Aires: Ministry of Health.

Munné M (1996). *A court and a hospital. Two agencies of social control. A psycho-sociological analysis of the social representations on alcohol and drugs in Argentina,* Paper presented at the 22nd Annual Alcohol Epidemiology Symposium of the Kettil Bruun Society, Edinburgh, Scotland, June 3-7.

Munné, M. (1999). *Alcohol and domestic violence: exploring the links and myths.* Paper presented at the 25th Annual Alcohol Epidemiology Symposium of the Kettil Bruun Society for Social and Epidemiological Research on Alcohol. Montreal, Canada. May 31-June 4.

Munné, M. (2001a). *Young people from at risk groups and alcohol in Argentina: an exploratory study* Paper presented at. International conference Youth Cultures and Subcultures: functions and patterns of drinking and drug use. Skarpö, Sweden, April 23-26.

Munné, M (2001b). Drinking in tango lyrics: an approach to myths and meanings of drinking in Argentinian culture. *Contemporary Drug Problems,* **28**, 415-439.

Munné, M (2003). *Alcohol and the economic crisis in Argentina: Recent findings.* Paper presented at 29th Annual Alcohol Epidemiology Symposium of the Kettil Bruun Society for Social and Epidemiological Research on Alcohol, Krakow, Poland, June.

Mustonen, H, et al. (2000) *Relationships of drinking behaviour, gender, and age with reported alcohol-related problems in Namibia.* Paper presented at 26th Annual Alcohol Epidemiology Symposium of the Kettil Bruun Society for Social and Epidemiological Research on Alcohol, Oslo, Norway, June5-9.

Necci, S. (1990). Que saben las familias porteñas sobre las drogas (What Argentinian families know about drugs). *Revista de Prevención, Salud y Sociedad,* **3**, 25-35.

Partanen, J. (1991). *Sociability and intoxication: alcohol and drinking in Kenya, Africa, and the Modern World.* Helsinki: Finnish Foundation For Alcohol Studies (Vol. 39).

Riley, L. & Marshall, M. (eds.) (1999). *Alcohol and Public Health in 8 Developing Countries.* Geneva: World Health Organisation.

Room, R, (1996), Alcohol consumption and social harm: Conceptual issues and historical perspectives. *Contemporary Drug Problems,* **23**, 373-388.

Room. R. (2001). New findings in alcohol epidemiology In: Nina Rehm with Robin Room and Griffith Edwards. *Alcohol in the European Region Consumption, Harm and Policies.* Copenhagen: WHO Regional Office for Europe (pp. 35-42).

Room, R. et al. (2002.) *Alcohol in Developing Societies: A Public Health Approach.* Helsinki: Finnish Foundation For Alcohol Studies (in collaboration with World Health Organisation).

SADA (2004). *Estudio de drogas en el conurbano bonaerense.* (Study of drugs in the province of Buenos Aires). La Plata: SADA (Secretaría de atención de las adicciones de la Provincia de Buenos Aires). (Secretary for the assistance of addictions in the province of Buenos Aires).

SEDRONAR (1994). (Secretaría de Programación para la Prevención de la Drogadicción y Lucha contra el Narcotráfico) *Investigación intrahospitalaria sobre consumo de drogas.* (intrahospital survey of the consumption of drugs) Buenos Aires: SEDRONAR.

SEDRONAR (2004). *Informe preliminar. Segundo estudio nacional sobre el consumo de sustancias psicoactivas Argentina 2004.* (Preliminary Report. Second national study of the use of psychoactive substances. Argentina 2004) Buenos Aires: SEDRONAR.

Tendencias Económicas (2002). *La economía argentina (The Argentinian economy).* Buenos Aires: Tendencias Económicas.

Verruno, C. et al. (1995). *Análisis del consumo del alcohol a partir de los datos de producción* (Analysis of the consumption of alcohol departing from the production data) Buenos Aires: PROESA.

Wilsnack. R. et al (2000). Gender differences in alcohol consumption and adverse drinking consequences: cross-cultural patterns. *Addiction* 95 (2), 251-265.

World Health Organisation (1999). *Global Status Report on Alcohol*. Geneva: World Health Organization.

World Health Organization (2000). *International Guide for Monitoring Alcohol Consumption and Related Harm*. Geneva: World Health Organization.

WHOSIS (2004) (WHO statistical information system) *Global Alcohol Database*. http//www.who.int/alcohol/alcohol_apc_data.

CHAPTER 3

DIFFERENCES IN DRINKING PATTERNS BETWEEN MEN AND WOMEN IN BRAZIL

FLORENCE KERR-CORRÊA, ANDREA M. HEGEDUS, LUZIA A. TRINCA,
ADRIANA M. TUCCI, LIGIA R. S. KERR-PONTES,
ALESSANDRA F. SANCHES & TRICIA M.F. FLORIPES

INTRODUCTION

Early studies on drinking and drinking patterns focused primarily on men; however literature has expanded to include studies on women. More recently with the growth of international collaboration, there is an increasing body of literature that examines the differences in drinking between men and women in different cultures and contexts.

The study of alcohol use and gender across cultures is important for several reasons. According to Wilsnack and Wilsnack (1997), gender differences in alcohol consumption are based on the ways each culture sees male and female roles. Consequently, gender differences in drinking vary according to cultural differences in social roles. Also, differences in alcohol use reflect the broader behavioural aspects of gender roles. A better understanding of why men and women have different drinking patterns can give insight into the fundamental characteristics of gender roles, and how these roles may change or resist change. Finally, understanding gender differences in alcohol use may prevent costly biases in how societies attempt to control or reduce alcohol related problems. Women's alcohol problems have often been neglected, being either viewed as not needing or deserving help, or resulting in punishment rather than treatment. On the other hand, men frequently regard their own drinking as "normal" until it impairs their behaviour and social relations.

One recent review of 16 general population surveys from 10 countries (Wilsnack et al., 2000) found that while there was little difference between women and men in the probability of current drinking versus abstaining, men always exceeded women in drinking frequency and quantity and in rates of heavy drinking episodes and adverse drinking consequences. Consistently, women were more likely than men to be lifetime abstainers. The authors concluded that gender differences in drinking might be biologically influenced. However, substantial variations between countries in the magnitude of these differences could suggest that sociocultural factors have a strong influence. Many countries have studied women's alcohol use and gender specificities; these include the Netherlands (Neve et al., 1996), Mexico (Medina-Mora, 1994), Czech Republic (Kubicka et al., 1995), the Nordic countries (Haavio-Mannila, 1989), and Nigeria (Ikuesan, 1994). Literature has shown that the consequences of patterns of use can impact drinkers as much or more than drinking levels and symptom severity (Marlatt et al., 1998). In the Federal Republic of Brazil, Almeida-Filho et al. (2004) analysed hazardous alcohol use by gender in a Northeast city of Brazil. They defined hazardous drinking as daily or weekly binge drinking plus episodes of drunkenness or frequent drunkenness (at least once a week). They found that 56% of respondents admitted to drinking. The overall 12-month prevalence of high-risk drinking was 7%, and was six times more prevalent in males than females (about 13% compared to 2.4%). A positive association to high-risk drinking was also found with education and social class, but not with ethnicity. Being male and of higher socio-economic status were associated with increased odds of high-risk drinking.

Hypotheses regarding gender differences in alcohol use stem primarily from the biological and socio-cultural aspects (Graham et al., 1998; Wilsnack et al., 2000). Biologically, the same amount of alcohol consumed by a man and a woman of the same weight will produce a higher blood alcohol concentration in the woman. There are several reasons for this, including women's lower body water content (Jones and Jones, 1976), differences in alcohol dehydrogenase (Frezza et al., 1990), metabolism (NIAAA, 2000), and hormone levels (Gavaler et al., 1993). Interacting with these biological factors are socio-cultural influences in drinking behaviour that have recently received considerable attention in literature. Areas of interest, other than cross-cultural genders differences in alcohol use patterns, include abstinence, intoxication, and related sexual behaviours (Wilsnack et al., 2000).

The repressive "war on drugs" policies exported by the United States were adapted by Brazil in the 1980's to primarily combat marijuana and cocaine use. Twenty years later, the number of users still continues to grow, illustrating the inadequacy of relying upon repressive measures. Alcohol-related problems are greater than drug-related problems in Brazil, but health policies have been negligent when addressing them. In addition, there are substantial regional differences in economic status, access to healthcare, education, and cultural backgrounds within the country. All of these factors are reflected in the patterns and use of alcohol and in drug consumption. However, only a few studies in Brazil delineate these differences. This dearth of information opens the way to imported policies being adopted that are often inadequate in addressing Brazilian reality.

Alcohol use and its related problems are greater than those associated with illicit drugs. A Brazilian study of students (aged 12-18) in 1987 showed that about 75% had already used alcohol, 22% had smoked tobacco, but the number who had used marijuana and cocaine were considerably lower: 2.8% and 0.5% respectively (Galduróz et al., 1987). At the same time, alcohol was involved in 95% of hospital admissions in alcohol/drug units, while marijuana only accounted for 1.4% and cocaine 0.8% (Noto & Carlini, 1995).

Prevalence of alcohol abuse in Brazil varies across studies. Moreira et al. (1996) in Porto Alegre (southern Brazil) found that 9.3% of their sample was alcohol dependent, 15.5% were heavy drinkers, 12.3% drank daily, and 12.3% were abstainers. Another study in Salvador (northeastern Brazil) showed that 37% of drivers involved in traffic accidents were under the influence of alcohol (Nery-Filho et al., 1995). Carlini et al. (1989) found alcohol use among students to be 9.2% and Galduróz et al. (1997) found 15.0%. A survey of households in São Paulo State reported alcohol dependency as 10.9% in men and 2.5% in women (Galduróz et al., 2003). Another household survey that studied the 107 largest cities in Brazil (Carlini et al., 2002) found 17.1% of men and 5.7% of women to be alcohol dependent. These results show an increasing trend in alcohol abuse incidence between the end of 80's and more recently.

In Brazil, as in many other developing countries, there is a tendency to think about alcohol-related problems primarily in the extreme case of alcohol dependency. But studies have shown that there are larger and just as serious alcohol-related problems across the spectrum of drinking behaviours (Cahalan & Room, 1974). Important strategies that governments in various countries have been using to control alcohol-related problems are the regulation of alcohol pricing and taxation. Studies show that increasing alcohol taxation and cost results in decreased alcohol use and its related problems (Babor et al., 2003). Although regulation is easy to establish by law and can be supervised at low cost, the taxes and price of alcohol in Brazil are very low. The very low price of alcohol products in Brazil has contributed to the increase in alcohol consumption, primarily among young people (Carlini-Cotrim et al., 1989, 1990, 2002; Galduróz et al., 1994, 2003). The most popular alcoholic beverage in Brazil is "cachaça" or "pinga," a distilled beverage made from sugarcane. It is very cheap (less than one dollar per liter) and has a very high alcohol content (around 40%). While beer (mostly 4.5 to 5% in ethanol content) has the highest national consumption by sheer volume, "cachaça" is highest in terms of ethanol content and it accounts for 80% of all distilled beverage consumption in Brazil (Moreira et al., 1996).

In Brazil, there is an extremely tolerant attitude toward alcohol consumption. Federal law that regulates alcohol advertising in Brazil allows beverages with alcohol content lower than 13% to be considered as food. Therefore, beer can be advertised in prime time television slots and targeted at teenagers. Also, beer is not seen as an alcoholic beverage, in fact the general public accept it almost as a soft drink.

There are other important issues regarding alcohol consumption and its related problems in Brazil. Access to alcohol is relatively easy. The law that imposes a minimum age for purchasing alcohol (18 years) is not enforced. There are no laws that control operating hours of bars, regulate licenses to sell alcohol, or limit places where alcohol can be bought. The maximum blood alcohol concentration allowed for drivers is 0.06%, however in practice, there are not enough devices or police to enforce it.

Some countries use public health policies to restrict access to alcohol; these have had considerable impact in relation to road accidents (Babor et al., 2003). São Paulo State limited the supply of alcohol in the driving environment by banning sales in commercial facilities on or near state highways (DETRAN – SP, 2004). Despite almost no enforcement, there was a significant reduction in crashes causing injuries. This illustrates that such policies, while relatively simple and not consistently applied, can have an impact on drinking and driving behaviour.

There are few studies that document alcohol-related medical problems in Brazil. Mott et al. (1989) found that 93.6% of chronic pancreatitis patients in São Paulo city exhibited heavy alcohol use. Alcoholism was the main cause of chronic pancreatitis (Dani et al., 1990) and cirrhosis of the liver (Strauss et al., 1988). Lolio (1990) found a significant association between high arterial hypertension and heavy alcohol use in the urban population of Araraquara (a city of São Paulo state). In another study, Nappo (1996) reported that alcohol was the most common substance used in drug-related non-natural deaths in São Paulo city. In a household survey in São Paulo State, Noto et al. (2004) evaluated the cases of household interpersonal violence and the consumption of alcohol and other drugs. They found that when violence was reported, 52% of perpetrators were intoxicated by alcohol.

In summary, Brazil has no specific restrictions on the off-premise sale of alcoholic beverages, no licensing system for alcohol beverage production, no control of retail sales and licensing, no health warning labels, no enforcement of advertising restrictions, and sponsorship restrictions are minimal (WHO, 2004).

This report is a further analysis of Brazilian data from the GENACIS project (Kerr-Corrêa et al., 2003), a multinational project that aims to compare patterns of alcohol use/abuse between the genders in different contexts in several countries (Bloomfield et al., 2005; Wilsnack & Wilsnack, 2002). This chapter discusses the results of administering the GENACIS questionnaire in a Brazilian regional sample in terms of gender differences in drinking patterns, ranging from abstinence to problem and heavy drinking.

METHODS

SETTING

Located in central São Paulo State in Southeast Brazil, Botucatu has 108,306 inhabitants. It is predominantly urban (96.2%), and has an annual growth rate of 1.64% (IBGE, 2004). About 98.8% of households are connected to the public water supply and sewage system; this is approximately three times the national rate and double the general Southeast Brazilian rate — the richest area of the country (IBGE, 2004). The municipality has 4,000 enterprises and the economy is commerce and service industry based; no single activity prevails.

SAMPLING

The GENACIS questionnaire was included as a component in a morbidity and service use survey conducted by UNESP (Universidade Estadual Paulista) Public Health Department. A stratified sample, representative of socio-economic and educational levels, was drawn from Botucatu, a São Paulo State town, and included those over 17 years old. Each stratum was composed by sector census (IBGE, 2004) and respondents were selected using cluster-sampling schemes. The sampling unit was family households, including apartments and single dwellings; student housing and commercial buildings were not included. Interviews were conducted in as private a setting as possible. More than one person per household could be interviewed. The final sample included 740 individuals who underwent face-to-face interviews in 2001 and 2002. Overall, approximately 5.8% refused to participate and some preferred not to respond to a few questions, primarily in the violence/intimacy section.

PROCEDURE

Female interviewers, experienced in population surveys, were given advanced training regarding the GENACIS questionnaire by the first author, and administered all measures used in this study. This advanced training included information specific to alcohol and drinking behaviour (e.g., antecedents and consequences, problem behaviour, and binge drinking), and violence, sexual, and intimacy questions. Interviewers were supervised monthly throughout the year to resolve any questions that arose, control for interview bias and drift, and address issues regarding the sensitivity of some of the questions in this culture. Only female interviewers were hired because, traditionally, females have easier access to other people's houses in Brazil, especially when intimate questions are asked.

MEASURES

GENACIS QUESTIONNAIRE ON GENDER, ALCOHOL AND CULTURE

The Genacis questionnaire was developed by an international group of investigators who were interested in the comparison of drinking patterns between the genders in different contexts and cultures. It has been used in a multinational study that includes a Brazilian component. The version used in this study consisted of a core questionnaire of 59 items, with sections on: demographics; work experiences; social networks; drinking variables — including quantity/frequency; context; family history of alcohol use; expectancies when using; and several consequences of alcohol use – and on intimate relationships and sexuality, violence and victimization, and health and lifestyle, including illicit and prescription drug use.

The questionnaire was translated into a Brazilian Portuguese version. The translation process included several steps: a) Forward translation by several psychiatrists, who were bilingual; b) Back translation by a native English professional translator who has been living in Brazil for several years; and c) Twenty pilot interviews conducted to identify and correct wording problems.

Self Report Questionnaire (SRQ)

This measure is a 20 item, self-assessment of mental health (Harding et al., 1980) that has been validated in Brazil by Mari and Willians (1986). A score above 7 is considered to indicate high risk of having a mental disorder.

Alcohol Consumption Variables

All alcohol consumption (e.g., beer, wine, liquor, etc.) was standardized to one drink of 12g of ethanol, which is the size of the average drink in Brazil.

Respondents were considered to be **abstinent** when they reported not drinking at all in the past year. **Light infrequent drinking** (LD) was defined as drinking at least one, but less than three drinks per occasion, once or less than once a month in the last 12 months. **Light frequent drinking** (LF) was defined as reporting at least one, but less than 3, drinks per occasion weekly or more in the last year. **Moderate infrequent drinking** (MI) was defined as drinking at least three, but less than four drinks per occasion, once or less than once a month in the last 12 months. **Moderate frequent drinking** (MF) was defined as drinking at least three, but less than four drinks per occasion weekly or more in the last year. **Heavy infrequent drinking** (HI) was defined as drinking at least 5 drinks per occasion once or less than once a month in the last 12 months. **Heavy frequent drinking** (HD) was defined as drinking at least 5 drinks per occasion, weekly or more in the last year, but not qualifying for the problem drinking category. **Problem drinking** (PD) was defined by: 1) as drinking at least 5 drinks per occasion weekly or more in the last year *and* at least one of the following; 2) one negative consequence (e.g., legal, clinical, psychiatric, familial, work) at any time in the last 12 months; 3) any dependence criterion. All drinking categories were mutually exclusive.

STATISTICAL ANALYSES

Association between alcohol use and each of the several socio-demographic variables was investigated by the chi-square test or the Fisher's exact test. Logistic regression analysis was employed to explore the strength of the possible explanatory variables to predict drinking in two models, one for predicting drinking versus non-drinking (abstainers) and the other for predicting heavy drinking versus non-heavy drinking. Here heavy drinking was a category composed by heavy (infrequent or frequent) and problem drinking. For this last model abstainers were excluded from the analysis. In each case a backward variable selection procedure was performed to select the most important predictors (a significance level of 0.15 was used to delete a variable from the model). For the first logistic analysis (drinking vs. non-drinking) the variables considered in the model were: total family income, age, marital status, religion, education level (compared to post secondary education), paid work (compared to not paid work), tobacco use, positive family alcohol use history, friend's drinking problems, level of partner's drinking, marriage satisfaction, self assessment of physical and emotional health, and SRQ total score. For the second logistic analysis (heavy vs. non-heavy use) all these variables, including effect of drinking on talking to the partner about feelings or problems and finding it easier to open up with other people under the influence of alcohol. These analyses were performed separately for males and females and were conducted using SAS (SAS, 1996).

ETHICAL CONSIDERATIONS

The Ethical Committee on Research of Botucatu Medical School, UNESP, approved this project on 4 April 2001.

RESULTS

SOCIOECONOMIC DATA

Table 1 shows the main socio-economic characteristics of the sample. Of the 740 interviewees 372 (50.3%) were male (age 17 to 93, mean 50 ± 21.09) and 368 (49.7%) were female (age 17 to 97, mean 50.9 ± 16.5). Most were married or living in a common law marriage (73.4%). About 32.2% of the respondents had at least eight years of education (14.4% of which had a college education), and 3.7% were illiterate. Regarding ethnicity, the majority of the interviewees were Caucasian (84.6%), followed by Mulatto (10.7%), Black (3.5%), and Asian (0.5%). About 70.8% were Catholic, 15% Evangelical/Protestant, 5.4% Kardecist or other religious faiths, and 6.2%

were agnostics/atheists.. Family income for about 45% was seven times or more the minimum wage (one minimum wage = U$100 per month), with around 15% receiving less than 3 times the minimum wage. As many women as men reported total family income above 7 times the minimum wage (48.8% vs. 44.6 %; p=0.275). Approximately 80.6% were in paid work, no males reported doing housework, 7.3% were students, and 3.5% were unemployed. For females about 17.1% were housewives who did not earn money. Except for household chores, socio-economic data was similar between genders.

TABLE 1. Socio-demographic characteristics of the Brazilian sample (%)

Characteristics	Male (n=372; 50.3%)	Female (n=368; 49.7%)	Total (n=740)
Age (mean SD)	50.3±21.09	50.9±16.5	
Education			
Illiterate	4.3	3.0	3.7
< 8 years	63.2	65.1	64.1
>/= 8 years	32.5	31.9	32.2
Religion			
Agnostic/Atheist	8.3	4.1	6.2
Catholic	69.6	72.0	70.8
Evangelical/Protestant	15.3	14.7	15.0
Kardecist	2.7	3.8	3.3
Other	1.3	3.0	2.1
No information	2.8	2.4	2.6
Marital status			
Married	62.3	60.5	61.4
Common law	12.1	11.8	12.0
Widowed	4.6	7.1	5.8
Divorced	9.2	6.8	8.0
Single	11.9	13.7	12.8
Family income (1 minimum wage = U$100/month)			
</= 2 minimum wages	18.0	12.8	15.4
3-6 minimum wages	35.8	37.5	36.6
>/=7 minimum wages	43.3	47.8	45.6
No information	2.9	1.9	2.4
Ethnic group			
Caucasian	83.3	85.6	84.6
Black	4.6	2.5	3.5
Mulatto	10.2	11.4	10.7
Asian	0.5	0.5	0.5
No information	1.3	0.0	0.7
Occupation			
Paid work	87.2	74.5	80.6
Student	8.5	6.0	7.3
Housewife	0.0	17.1	8.6
Unemployed	4.4	2.5	3.5

TABLE 2. Abstinence and drinking patterns among current drinkers during the last 12 months by gender and age group

Drinking category	Male (n=372)				Female (n=368)				Total (N=740)
	18 to 34 (n=115)	35 to 49 (n=70)	50 to 64 (n=63)	∅ 65 (n=124)	18 to 34 (n=99)	35 to 49 (n=57)	50 to 64 (n=71)	∅ 65 (n=141)	n (%)
Abstainers	42.6	45.7	50.8	43.6	44.4	57.9	45.1	43.3	337(45.5)
Infrequent light	19.1	11.4*	20.6	17.7	17.2	22.8*	15.5	21.3	136(18.4)
Frequent light	18.3	7.2	12.7	21.8	20.2	10.5	21.1	22.7	134(18.1)
Infrequent moderate	0.0	0.0	0.0	0.0	1.0	0.0	0.0	0.0	1 (0.1)
Frequent moderate	7.0	8.6	6.4	7.3	6.1	1.8	12.7	5.7	51 (6.9)
Infrequent heavy	3.5	5.7	4.8	4.0	7.1	0.0	1.4	0.7	25 (3.4)
Frequent heavy	4.4	8.6	1.6	3.2	2.0	3.5	0.0	3.6	25 (3.4)
Problem drinker	5.2	12.9*	3.2	2.4	2.0	3.5*	4.2	2.8	31 (4.2)

*p<0.05

DRINKING PATTERNS

Table 2 shows the percentages of abstainers and current drinker drinking patterns stratified by age and gender. Abstinence was high in all age groups in both sexes. Unsurprisingly, the only significant difference between genders was for light infrequent drinking (twice as common among women) and problem drinking (almost four times as common among men) aged 35 to 49. As we did not find any men and found just one woman classified as a moderate infrequent drinker, the moderate drinkers were combined.

Table 3 shows that abstinence was more prevalent among Christians of both genders. Caucasian, more educated, and those on higher income were more likely to be drinkers (compared to abstainers). Marital status had different associations for men and women: divorced women and those living in common law were more likely to be drinkers, while men who were divorced or living in common law were more likely to be heavy frequent or problem drinkers. Unemployment showed the highest rates of problem drinking for both genders. More Black and Mulatto women were found to be light frequent drinkers. Furthermore, among housewives there were no heavy frequent or problem drinkers and they had the highest rates of abstention. The opposite was found for women who had a job as they were more likely to be drinkers. Female students were more likely to be abstainers or moderate drinkers than males.

Table 4 shows the results of the logistic regression for predicting current drinking vs. abstention according to gender. For women, having a heavy drinking partner, being in paid work, and being unemployed were

TABLE 3.   Socio-demographic data and alcohol use patterns in the last 12 months by gender

Variable	Male								Female							
	Total	Abst ainer	Infre quent	Freq uent light	Mod erate light	Infre quent heavy	Freq uent heavy	Pro blem drin ker	Total	Abst ainer	Infre quent	Freq uent light	Mod erate light	Infre quent heavy	Freq uent heavy	Pro blem drin ker
	N	%	%	%	%	%	%	%	N	%	%	%	%	%	%	%
Religion																
Catholic	259	45.2	15.1	17.0	8.1	3.9	5.0	5.8	265	47.9	20.0	17.4	6.4	2.3	2.3	3.8
Evangelical	57	47.4	26.3	8.8	5.3	5.3	1.8	5.3	54	50.0	16.7	18.5	7.4	5.6	1.9	0.0
Agnostic	31	32.3	22.6	25.8	6.5	3.2	3.2	6.5	15	26.7	13.3	40.0	13.3	0.0	6.7	0.0
Other	15	46.7	20.0	20.0	0.0	13.3	0.0	0.0	25	28.0	28.0	36.0	4.0	0.0	4.0	0.0
Education																
≤ 7 years	51	58.2	12.8	13.3	5.1	2.6	2.6	5.6	200	58.5	14.5	17.5	3.5	2.0	1.5	2.5
8 to 11 years	125	33.6	20.0	18.4	11.2	7.2	5.6	4.0	112	33.9	22.3	22.3	10.7	2.7	3.6	4.5
∅ 12 years	51	21.6	29.4	23.5	5.9	3.9	7.8	7.8	55	25.5	30.9	23.6	10.9	3.6	3.6	1.8
Family income																
≤ 2 min. wages	67	52.2	14.9	16.4	6.0	1.5	3.0	6.0	47	53.2	12.8	27.7	2.1	2.1	2.1	0.0
3-6 min. wages	133	46.6	17.3	14.3	6.8	6.8	2.3	6.0	138	50.0	17.4	17.4	6.5	2.2	2.9	3.6
∅7 min. wages	161	40.4	19.3	18.0	8.1	3.8	6.2	4.4	176	40.3	23.3	19.9	8.6	2.8	1.7	3.4
Occupation																
Paid work	320	46.3	17.5	16.3	7.2	3.1	4.4	5.3	274	41.2	20.4	23.7	5.8	2.6	2.9	3.3
Unemployed	16	43.8	18.8	6.3	12.5	6.3	0.0	12.5	9	22.2	11.1	11.1	33.0	0.0	11.1	11.1
Housewife	0	-	-	-	-	-	-	-	63	76.2	11.1	11.1	1.6	0.0	0.0	0.0
Student	31	22.6*	19.4*	25.8	6.5*	16.1	6.5	3.2	22	31.8*	31.8*	0.0	22.8*	9.1	0.0	4.6
Ethnic group																
Caucasian	312	43.0	18.0	19.2	6.1	4.5	5.1	4.2	317	45.1	21.1	20.8	5.4	2.8	2.2	2.5
Black/ Mulatto	55	52.7	16.4	1.8*	14.6	3.6	0.0	10.9	51	52.9	7.8	13.7*	15.7	0.0	3.9	5.9
Maritalstatus																
Married	231	43.3	16.5	18.2	8.7	4.3	4.3	4.8	221	46.2	19.0	19.9	6.8	1.8	2.7	3.6
Common law	45	33.3	28.9*	8.9*	11.1	0.0	4.4	13.3	43	44.2	11.6*	25.6*	11.7	2.3	4.7	0.0
Widowed	17	35.3	23.5	17.7	5.9	11.8	5.9	0.0	26	42.3	23.1	19.2	0.0	7.7	3.9	3.9
Divorced	34	47.1*	8.8*	23.5	2.9	5.9	8.8	2.9	25	24.0*	28.0*	28.0	8.0	8.0	0.0	4.0
Single	44	68.2	15.9	6.8	0.0	4.6	0.0	4.6	50	60.0	22.0	10.00	6.0	0.0	0.0	2.0

* p<0.05

associated with drinking. For men, having friends who drank alcohol, low SRQ scores, smoking (tobacco), and marital status (married, common law or widow) were associated with drinking. For both men and women, drinking seemed to increase with level of education: those with eight or more years of education were more likely to drink than those with less than eight years of education.

Table 5 shows results of the logistic regression analyses for predicting heavy drinking (heavy infrequent, heavy frequent, or problem drinker). Drinking alone was associated with heavy and/or problem drinking for

TABLE 4. Logistic regression model for predicting drinking (1=drinkers; 0=non-drinkers) in the last 12 months

Variable	Male Odds ratio*	(95% CI)	Female Odds ratio*	(95% CI)
Marital status				N.S
Married	2.20	(1.01-4.83)		
Common law	3.16	(1.16-8.58)		
Widowed	4.14	(1.06-16.19)		
Divorced	2.10	(0.73-6.08)		
Single	1.00			
Education				
12+ years	6.19	(2.81-13.66)	3.38	(1.62-7.03)
8 to 11 years	2.41	(1.44-4.04)	2.53	(1.46-4.37)
Less than 8 years	1.00		1.00	
Tobacco use				
Yes	2.41	(1.40-4.15)		NS
Family alcohol history				
Yes	2.30	(1.34-3.96)	3.26	(1.80-5.90)
Friends use of alcohol				
Yes	3.64	(1.72-7.70)		NS
SRQ	2.13	(1.18-3.86)		
Low				
Occupation		NS		
Student			2.91	(0.88-9.62)
Paid work			4.16	(2.02-8.54)
Unemployed			10.96	(1.86-64.74)
Housewife			1.00	
Partner heavy drinker		NS	2.93	(1.16-7.38)
Yes			2.93	(1.16-7.38)

Note: significant (p<0.05) results are shown when at least one result for the predictor was significant.
* Adjusted to all the other variables in the model.

TABLE 5. Logistic regression model for being a heavy drinker (infrequent, frequent and problem) among current drinkers (1=heavy drinkers; 0=non heavy drinkers)

Variable	Male Odds ratio*	(95% CI)	Female Odds ratio*	(95% CI)
Age				
65	0.67	(0.28-1.61)		NS
50 to 64	0.80	(0.27-2.34)		
35 to 49	3.10	(1.29-7.49)		
18 to 34	1.00			
Tobacco use				
Yes	1.95	(0.99-3.84)		NS
Drinks alone				
Yes		NS	3.26	(1.42-7.47)

Note: Significant (p<0.05) results are shown when at least one result for the predictor was significant.
* Adjusted to all the other variables in the model.

women. For men, smoking and being between 35 and 49 years of age were associated with heavy and/or problem drinking.

DISCUSSION

This study used a Brazilian version of a questionnaire that had already been developed as a standardized, culturally sensitive measure of drinking and its consequences. Results from this stratified, urban, representative sample of 740 subjects from a town of 108,306 inhabitants showed that abstinence was common: about 45% of men and 46% of women during the last 12 months. At the low drinking levels, women and men had very similar drinking patterns. The women demonstrated changes in their socio-cultural roles in that they were frequently working outside the home, had good incomes, and more access to alcohol. As their roles became more similar to men's, so did their drinking patterns. Caucasians, the more educated, and people with higher incomes, were less likely to be abstainers. As expected for a Latin American country, religious affiliation (Catholics and Evangelical/Protestants) seemed an important reason for abstinence in this region.

For women, the only risk factor for heavy drinking was drinking alone. For men, smoking and being between 35 and 49 were associated with heavy drinking.

While biological differences between women and men are important factors in the determination of alcohol use, socio-cultural factors also seem to play an important role. This study found that several important socio-cultural variables had an impact on gender differences in drinking, including demographic characteristics (e.g., employment, education, marital status, etc.), and social roles. These differences were also examined in terms of different drinking patterns.

Overall, this regional sample differed somewhat from those described in other studies. Only 4.7% of the Brazilian population has 12 or more years of formal education and about 20.0% are illiterate compared to Botucatu, which presents 14.3% and 3.6%, respectively (www.datasus.gov.br). Even compared to the Southeast region, where Botucatu is located, this town fares better (9.1% and 8.4%, respectively). Carmo et al. (2003) have discussed this epidemiological transition in developing countries such as Brazil. Compared to developed countries where decreases in infectious and parasitic diseases and increases in chronic-degenerative diseases, accidents, and violence-related health events are due to improvements in social and economic conditions, in Brazil, these trends are present in the context of extreme complexity and social inequality. Brazil presents a paradoxical situation, where economic indicators (15th world economy in 2004) are incompatible with social indicators. As a whole, all Brazilian regions are improving, but at drastically different levels, rates, and velocity. Botucatu is an example of this phenomenon: it is a relatively small university town that has all its indicators (water supply, sewage, health system, educational achievement, employment, and salaries, including good jobs for women, among others) well above regional and national levels.

Because the sample was drawn from this town, with its long history of good medical services, the respondents were older, Caucasian, married or living in common law, and most women worked outside the home and earned good salaries. This may be seen as a major limitation to this study. Therefore, the results are not generalizable in that it was a stable, middle-class sample with women who functioned outside the more traditional roles found in other areas of Brazil. However, it was conducted over one year, stratified by neighbourhood, and representative of the socio-economical-educational level of this community. It should be seen as a study at one end of the socio-economic continuum in a country undergoing major social and economical transitions, which shows that when socio-cultural factors and social roles change, drinking differences between the genders tend to diminish.

This study tried to examine differences in drinking levels between women and men. The same amount of alcohol consumed by a woman and a man of the same weight will produce a higher blood alcohol concentration in women (Jones & Jones, 1976). Despite this discrepancy in physiological alcohol effects, many surveys use the same definitions of drinking levels for women and men. Use of gender-specific drinking measures that take into consideration female-male differences in body weight and body water content substantially reduces gender differences in reported alcohol consumption (Graham et al, 1998; York & Welte, 1994; Wilsnack et al, 1997). Because of the small number of people in the heavy and/or problem drinker's categories, we could not conduct separate analyses for different levels of drinking. However, we could find risk factors for drinking in both genders.

In this sample, abstinence levels were high, about 45% for both women and men. In general, levels of drinking, quantity, and frequency were similar between genders, and were predominantly light in pattern. Interestingly, in the older age group, we also found no differences between men and women. Nevertheless, when examining drinking at higher levels and different age groups, gender differences were more evident. There were more men than women problem drinkers in the 35-49 age group. This corresponds with our clinical experience in the same region, where there are substantially more men in treatment in this age range than women (Simão et al 2002).

Binge drinking, defined as 5 or more drinks per occasion (Wechsler et al., 1994) is a pattern of alcohol use associated with increased physical and emotional harm, including violence, accidents, unplanned pregnancy, unprotected sex, STD, and HIV. It is frequently found among men in most countries (Wilsnack et al., 2000). We consistently found more heavy drinking men than women, but this was not statistically significant. The sampling procedure may in part explain the lower prevalence of heavy drinking in single people, as it excluded most university students living in town.

The main predictors of a woman being a drinker (instead of an abstainer) were indicators of access to alcohol: these were higher education, having a partner who is a heavy drinker, and working outside the home for pay and/or considering herself as unemployed (or basically a worker, not a housewife). It is important to say that they were mostly light, not even moderate, drinkers. We only had 29 women who were in the heavy or problem drinker categories. It is a pattern frequently found in the literature on drinking when you have access, either through money or a partner who is a heavy drinker, and probably have alcoholic beverages available (and company) at home to drink. Using similar methodology as this study, it has been shown that women in several countries with higher status jobs and better education were more likely to drink (Gmel et al., 2000). Both clinical studies and general population surveys have found strong similarities between women's and their partner's drinking levels (Corbett et al., 1991; Demers et al., 1999; Hammer & Vaglum, 1989; Jacob & Bremer, 1986; Roberts & Leonard, 1997). Other studies have found that men have a stronger influence on their women's drinking pattern than vice versa (Wilsnack & Wilsnack, 1990).

The significant effect of a family history of alcoholism on the development of alcohol abuse has also been reported in several studies (Chassin et al., 1993; 1999, Sher et al., 1991). In this study, risk factors in both genders for drinking were higher education and a family history of an alcohol problem. Some studies have found the same traits among abstainers: lower incomes, lower level of education and older ages (ICAP, 2000).

None of these factors was important for heavy and/or problem drinkers, which only were associated with an indicator of alcohol dependence, i.e, drinking alone, as expected for women. For men, smoking and being aged 35 to 49 yeas were associated with heavy drinking.

In general, women in this sample could be seen as less conservative and less traditional than regional or national populations if they worked for pay, outside their homes or consider themselves as unemployed as opposed to housewives. As a result, the drinking pattern of working women was more equivalent to men, as were their social roles. Surprisingly we found not even one heavy or problem drinker among housewives, probably due to the small sample size.

Similar changes in drinking and sexual behaviour found recently in literature are also related to new social roles for women. Women in this study had higher rates of employment and income compared to other neighbourhoods in this area, with less abstinence, easier access to alcohol and higher rates of drinking (Kerr-Corrêa et al., 2003), Women's drinking has often been socially more restricted than men's out of the fear that drinking may more adversely affect women's social behaviour and responsibilities (Blume, 1997). Other authors have found that women's intoxication reduces social control of their sexuality, making them either more sexually uninhibited or more sexually vulnerable (Gomberg, 1982;

Stewart, 1992; Purcell, 1994). Traditionally, women's drinking has been discouraged or concealed because it was incompatible with domestic roles, and might interfere with social control over family relationships and public behaviour (Ikuesan, 1994; Purcell, 1994; Warner, 1997).

If gender differences in alcohol use have a socio-cultural basis, such as women's roles becoming similar to men's, women and men's drinking behaviours would be expected to converge. Some evidence of this has been reported in the past (Hammer & Vaglum, 1989; Mercer & Khavari, 1990; Saelan et al., 1992). Nevertheless, other researchers have found persistent gender differences, both in general adult populations (Bell et al., 1984; Midanik & Clark, 1994; Neve et al., 1996), university students, and young adult samples (Temple, 1987; Perkins, 1992; Johnston et al., 1994). This is a critical area of study that requires further investigation.

For men, low SRQ scores, friend's alcohol abuse, marital status (married, common law or widowed), level of education, and tobacco use were associated with drinking. The association between smoking and alcohol consumption has been well established in clinical and non-clinical populations (Henningfield et al., 1990; Istvan & Matazarro, 1984). Smokers are more likely to drink alcohol and drink higher quantity than nonsmokers (Zacny, 1990).

Another study in Brazil (Almeida-Filho et al., 2004) found that marriage or living with a partner was a protective factor for drinking in both genders. However, in this study we found the opposite result in men: being single was a protective factor, contrary to our expectations. This may be explained by the higher mean age of the sample and exclusion of most university students, as not living with their families (but in fraternities, shared houses and dormitories) they were not considered as living in households for sampling purposes.

In this survey, drinking alone was the only risk factor independently associated with heavy drinking in women. Other studies have found that women are more likely to drink alone than men without meaning necessarily dependence (Robbins & Martin, 1993). Nevertheless, in this work, the association seems indicative of harmful use of alcohol.

In summary, men generally had a higher level of alcohol use than women, but both men and women showed very similar patterns in light alcohol use, especially when considering women who were working outside their homes for pay or defined themselves as unemployed. This may indicate that they are already changing their socio-cultural roles. As their social roles become more similar to men's, so do their drinking patterns. This finding did not hold for individuals aged 35-49 years, which may be due to the family responsibilities of women, and the more frequent binge and/or problem drinking in men. More studies, especially with larger and more representative samples, are needed to capture in detail gender differences in alcohol use patterns in this population.

ACKNOWLEDGEMENT

Support for this study was provided by FAPESP Grant (00/03150-6; 01/12807-9).

REFERENCES

Almeida-Filho, N., Lessa, I., Magalhães, L., Araújo, M. J., Aquino, E., Kawachi, I., James, S. A. (2004). Social determinants and patterns of alcohol consumption in Bahia, Brazil. *Revista de Saúde Pública*, **38**, 1-13.

Babor, T. F., Caetano, R., Casswell, S., Edwards, G, Giesbrecht, N. et al . (2003). *Alcohol: no ordinary commodity*. Oxford: Oxford University Press, 301p.

Bell, R., Havlicek, P.L., Roncek, D. W. (1984). Sex differences in the use of alcohol and tranquilizers: testing a role convergence hypothesis. *American Journal of Drug and Alcohol Abuse*, **10**, 551-561.

Bloomfield, K., Allamani, A., Beck, F., Bergmark, K.H., Csemy, L. et al (2005). *Gender, culture and alcohol problems: a multi-national study. Project final report*. Berlin, Germany: Institute for medical informatics, biometrics and epidemiology, Charité Universitätsmedizin Berlin.

Blume, S.B. (1997). Women and alcohol: issues in social policy. In: R.W. Wilsnack, S.C., Wilsnack, (eds.), *Gender and alcohol: individual and social perspectives*. New Brunswick, NJ: Rutgers Center of Alcohol Studies: 462-489.

Cahalan, R., Room, R. (1974). *Problem drinking among American men*. New Brunswuick, NJ: Rutgers Centre of Alcohol Studies.

Carlini-Cotrim, B., Carlini, E., Silva-Filho, A. R., Barbosa, M. T. S. (1989). O uso de drogas psicotrópicas por estudantes de primeiro e segundo graus da rede estadual, em dez capitais brasileiras, 1987. (The use of psychotropic drugs by first and second degree students at the state network, in ten Brazilian capital, 1987.) In: *Consumo de drogas psicotrópicas no Brasil, em 1987*. Centro de Documentação, Ministério da Saúde, Brasilia, DF, Série C: Estudos e Projetos **5**, 9-84.

Carlini, E.A., Carlini-Cotrim, B., Silva-Filho, A.R. , Barbosa, M. T. S. (1990). *II Levantamento nacional sobre o uso de psicotrópicos em estudantes de primeiro e segundo graus,1989. (II National psychotropic use survey in first and second degree students, 1989.)* Centro Brasileiro de Informações sobre Drogas Psicotrópicas, Departamento de Psicobiologia, Escola Paulista de Medicina, São Paulo, SP, Brazil.

Carlini, E. A., Galduróz, J. C., Noto, A. R., Nappo, S. A. (2002). *I Levantamento domiciliar sobre o uso de drogas psicotrópicas no Brasil: estudo envolvendo as 107 maiores cidades do país, 2001. (I National psychotropic drug use survey in Brazil: study in the 107 biggest cities in the country, 2001.)* São Paulo: CEBRID – Centro Brasileiro de Informações Sobre Drogas Psicotrópicas: UNIFESP, Universidade Federal de São Paulo.

Carmo, E. H., Barreto, M. L., Silva, J. B. (2003). Mudanças nos padrões de morbimortalidade da população brasileira: os desafios para o novo século. (Change in morbimortality patterns in the Brazilian population: challenges to the new century). *Epidemiologia e Serviços de Saúde*, **12**, 63-75.

Chassin L., Pillow, D.R., Curran P.J., Molina B.S., Barrera M. (1993). Relation of parental alcoholism to early adolescent substance use: a test of three mediating mechanisms. *Journal Abnormal of Psychology*, **102**, 3–19.

Chassin L., Pitts S.C., DeLucia C. (1999). The relation of adolescent substance use to young adult autonomy, positive activity involvement, and perceived competence. *Development of Psychopathology,* **11**, 915-932.

Corbett, K., Mora, J., Ames, G. (1991). Drinking patterns and drinking-related problems of Mexican–American husbands and wives. *Journal of Studies on Alcohol,* **52**, 215–223.

Dani, R., Mott, C. B., Guarita, D. R., Nogueira, C. E. (1990). Epidemiology and etiology of chronic pancreatitis in Brazil: a tale of two cities. *Pancreas,* **5**, 474-478.

Demers, A., Bisson, J., Palluy, J. (1999). Wives convergence with their husbands' alcohol use: Social conditions as mediators. *Journal of Studies on Alcohol,* **60**, 368–377.

DETRAN–SP Departamento Estadual de Trânsito (2004) Álcool e trânsito. (State Department of Traffic). Internet: http://www.detran.sp.gov.br/campanhas/alcool_transito/in_alcool_transito.html

Frezza, M., Di Padova, C., Pozzato, G., Terpin, M., Baraona, E., Lieber, C. S. (1990). High blood alcohol levels in women: the role of decreased alcohol dehydrogenase activity in first pass metabolism. *New England Journal of Medicine,* **322**, 95-99.

Galduróz, J. C. F., D'Almeida, V., Carvalho, V., Carlini, E. A. (1994). *III Levantamento sobre o uso de drogas entre estudantes de 1º e 2º graus em 10 capitais brasileiras, 1993. (III Psychotropic use survey among 1º and 2º degrees students in 10 Brazilian capitals, 1993).* Centro Brasileiro de Informações sobre Drogas Psicotrópicas, Departamento de Psicobiologia, Escola Paulista de Medicina, Universidade Federal de São Paulo, São Paulo, SP, Brazil.

Galduróz, J. C. F., Noto, A. R., Carlini, E. A. (1997). *IV Levantamento sobre o uso de drogas entre estudantes de 1o e 2o graus em 10 capitais brasileiras 1997. (IV Psychotropic use survey among 1º and 2º degrees students in 10 Brazilian capitals 1997.)* São Paulo; Universidade Federal de São Paulo. Centro Brasileiro de Informações sobre drogas psicotrópicas – CEBRID.

Galduróz, J. C. F., Noto, A. R., Nappo, S. A., Carlini, E. L. A. (2003). First household survey on drug abuse in São Paulo, Brazil, 1999: principal findings. *São Paulo Medical Journal,* **121**, 231-237.

Gavaler, J. S., Deal, S. R., Van Thiel, D. H., Arria, A. M., Allan, M. J. (1993). Alcohol and estrogen levels in postmenopausal women: The spectrum of effect. *Alcoholism: Clinical and Experimental Research,* **17**, 786–790.

Gmel, G., Bloomfield, K., Alhström, S., Choquet, M., Lecomte, T. (2000). Women's roles and women's drinking: a comparative study in four European countries. *Substance Abuse,* **21**, 249-264.

Gomberg, E. S. L. (1982). Historical and political perspectives on women and drug use. *Journal of Social Issues,* **38**, 9-23.

Graham, K., Wilsnack, R., Dawson, D., Vogeltanz, N. (1998). Should alcohol measure be adjusted for gender differences? *Addiction,* **93**, 1717-1727.

Haavio-Mannila, E. (ed., 1989). *Women, alcohol, and drugs in the Nordic countries.* Helsinki: Nordic Concil for Alcohol and Drug Research.

Hammer, T., Vaglum, P. (1989). The increase in alcohol consumption among women: a phenomenon related to accessibility or stress? A general population study. *British Journal of Addiction,* **84**, 764-775.

Harding, T. W., Arango, M. V., Baltazar, J., Climent, C. E., Ibrahim, H. H. A., Ignacio, L. L., Murthy, R. S., Wig, N. N. (1980). Mental Disorders in primary health care: a study of their frequency and diagnosis in four development countries. *Psychological Medicine*, **10**, 231-241.

Henningfield, J.E., Clayton, R., Pollin, W. (1990). Involvement of tobacco in alcoholism and illicit drug use. *British Journal of Addiction*, **85**, 279-91.

IBGE (Instituto Brasileiro de Geografia e Estatística www.ibge.gov.br), 2004.

Ikuesan, B. A. (1994). Drinking problems and the position of women in Nigeria. *Addiction*, **89**, 941-944.

Istvan, J., Matarazzo, J.D. (1984). Tobacco, alcohol, and caffeine use: a review of their interrelationships. *Psychological Bulletin*, **95**, 301-326.

International Center for Alcohol Policies (June 2000). *Who are the abstainers?* ICAP Reports 8.

Jacob, T., Bremer, D. A. (1986). Assortative mating among men and women alcoholics. *Journal of Studies on Alcohol*, **47**, 219–222.

Johnston, L. D., O'Malley, P. M., Bachman, J. G. (1994). *National survey results on drug use from the monitoring the future study*. Vol. II. College students and young adults, NIH Publication 94-3810 (Rockville, MD, National Institute on Drug Abuse).

Jones, B. M., Jones, M. K. (1976). Women and alcohol: Intoxication, metabolism and the menstrual cycle. In: Greenblatt M and Schuckit MA, eds. *Alcoholism Problems in Women and Children*. New York, NY: Grune , Stratton (pp. 103–136).

Kerr-Corrêa, F., Sanches, A. F., Trinca, L. A. , Lima, M. C. P. (2003). Gender, culture and problems associated with alcohol: preliminary analysis of the Brazilian part of a multinational study. *Annals of the 29th KBS Annual Meeting*, Krakow, Poland.

Kubicka, L.; Csemy, L.; Kozeny, J. (1995). Prague women's drinking before and after the 'velvet revolution' of 1989: a longitudinal study. *Addiction*, **90**, 1471-1478.

Lolio, C. A. (1990). The epidemiology of arterial hypertension. *Revista de Saúde Pública*, **24**, 425-432.

Mari, J., Willians, P. A. (1986). A validity study of a psychiatric screening questionnaire (SRQ-20) in primary care in the city of São Paulo. *British Journal of Psychiatry*, **148**, 23-26.

Marlatt, G. A., Baer, J. S., Kivlahan, D. R., Dimeff, L. A., Larimer, M. E., Quigley, L. A., Somers, J. M., Williams, E. (1998). Screening and brief intervention for high-risk college student drinkers: results from a 2-years follow-up assessment. *Journal of Consulting and Clinical Psychology*, **66**, 604-615.

Medina-Mora, E. (1994). Drinking and the oppression of women: the Mexican experience. *Addiction*, **89**, 958-960.

Mercer, P. W., Khavari, K. A. (1990). Are women drinking more like men? An empirical examination of the convergence hypothesis. *Alcoholism: Clinical and Experimental Research*, **14**, 461-466.

Midanik, L. T., Clark, W. B. (1994). The demographic distribution of U.S. drinking patterns in 1990: description and trends from 1984. *American Journal of Public Health*, **84**, 1218-1222.

Moreira, L. B., Fuchs, F. D., Moraes, R. S., Bredemeier, M., Cardozo, S., Fuchs, S. C., Victora, C. G. (1996). Alcoholic beverage consumption and associated factors in Porto Alegre, a southern Brazilian city: a population-based survey. *Journal of Studies on Alcohol*, **57**, 253-259.

Mott, C. B., Guarita, D. R., Coelho, M. E., Monteiro da Cunha, J. E., Machado, M. C., Bettarello A. (1989). Etiology of chronic pancreatitis in Sao Paulo: a study of 407 cases. *Revista do Hospital das Clinicas da Faculdade de Medicina de São Paulo*, **44**, 214-220.

National Institute on Alcohol Abuse and Alcoholism (2000). Alcohol and women: an overview. 10th Special report to the US congress and alcohol and health. US Department of Health and Human Services: 253-257.

Nery-Filho, A., Miranda, M., Miranda, M. G. (1995). Estudo da alcoolemia numa amostra de população urbana de Salvador. (Alcoholemy study in an urban sample from Salvador.) Paper presented at the International Meeting on Drug Use and Abuse, Salvador, Bahia, Brasil.

Neve, R., Drop, M., Lemmens, P., Swinkels, H. (1996). Gender differences in drinking behaviour in the Netherlands: convergence or stability? Addiction, 91, 357-373.

Nappo, S. A., Galduróz, J. C. F. (1996). Psychotropic drug-related deaths in São Paulo city, Brazil. In: Annals of the X World Congress of Psychiatry, Madrid, Spain, X World Congress of Psychiatry.

Noto, A. R., Carlini, E. A. (1995). Internações hospitalares provocadas por drogas: análise de sete anos consecutivos (1987-1993). (Hospital admissions caused by drugs: analysis of seven consecutive years (1987-1993)). Revista da Associação Brasileira de Psiquiatria-Asociacion Psiquiatrica de la America Latina, 17, 107-114.

Noto, A. R., Fonseca, A. M., Silva, E. A., Gálduroz, J. C. F. (2004). Violência domiciliar associada ao consumo de bebidas alcoólicas e de outras drogas: um levantamento no Estado de São Paulo. (Home violence associated to alcoholic beverage and others drugs consumption: a survey in São Paulo State). Jornal Brasileiro de Dependência Química, 5, 9-17.

Perkins, H. W. (1992). Gender patterns in consequences of collegiate alcohol abuse: a 10-year study of trends in an undergraduate population. Journal of Studies on Alcohol, 53, 458-462.

Purcell, N. (1994). Women and wine in ancient Rome. In: M. MacDonald (eds.). Gender, drink and drugs: 191-208. Providence, RI.

Roberts, L. J., Leonard, K. E. (1997). Gender differences and similarities in the alcohol and marriage relationship. In: R. W. Wilsnack, S. C. Wilsnack (eds.), Gender and alcohol: individual and social perspectives: 289–311. Piscataway, NJ7 Rutgers Center of Alcohol Studies.

Robbins, C. A., Martin, S. S. (1993). Gender, styles of deviance, and drinking problems. Journal of Health and Social Behavior, 34, 302–321.

Saelan, H., Moler, L., Koster, A. (1992). Alcohol consumption in a Danish cohort during 11 years, Scandinavian Journal of Social Medicine, 20, 87-93.

SAS (1996). Software release 6.12. SAS Institute Inc. Carey, NC, USA.

Snare, A. (1989). Women and control. In: E. Haavio-Mannila E (ed). Women, Alcohol, and Drugs in the Nordic Countries: 133-152. Helsinki: Nordic Council for Alcohol and Drug Research.

Sher K.J., Walitzer K.S., Wood P.K., Brent E.E. (1991). Characteristics of children of alcoholics: putative risk factors, substance use and abuse, and psychopathology. Journal of Abnormal Psychology, 100, 427-448.

Simão, M.O., Kerr-Corrêa, F., Dalben, I., Smaira, S.I. (2002). Alcoholic and men: a comparative study of social and familial and outcome. Revista Brasileira de Psiquiatria, 24, 121-129.

Stewart, M. (1992). "I can´t drink beer, I've just drunk water": alcohol, bodily substance and commensality among Hungarian rom. In: D. Gefou-Madianou (ed.), Alcohol, Gender, and Culture: 137-156. New York, N.Y.: Routledge.

Strauss, E., Lacet, C. M., Maffei, J. R. A., Silva, E. C., Fukushima, J., Gayotto, L., Carlos, C. (1988). Etiologia e apresentação da cirrose hepática em São Paulo:

análise de 200 casos (Etiology and clinical aspects of liver cirrhosis in Säo Paulo, Brazil: analysis of 200 cases). *Gastroenterologia Endoscópica Digestiva*, **7**, 119-23.

Temple, M. (1987). Alcohol use among male and female college students: has there been a convergence? *Youth and Society*, **19**, 44-72.

Warner, J. (1997). The sanctuary of sobriety: the emergence of temperance as a feminine virtue in Tudor and Stuart England. *Addiction*, **92**, 97-111.

Wechsler, H., Davenport, A., Dowdal, G., Moeykens, B. , Castillo, S. (1994). Health and behavioral consequences of binge drinking in college: A national survey of students at 140 campuses. *JAMA*, **272**, 1672-1677.

Wilsnack, S. C., Plaud, J. J., Wilsnack, R. W., Klassen, A. D. (1997). Sexuality, gender and alcohol use. In: R.W. Wilsnack, S.C. Wilsnack (eds). *Gender and alcohol: individual and social perspectives*. New Brunnswick, NJ: Rutgers Center of Alcohol Studies. Alcohol, culture, and social control monograph series 3.

Wilsnack, R. W., Wilsnack, S. C. (1997). *Gender and alcohol: Individual and social perspectives*. New Brunswick, NJ: Rutgers Center of Alcohol Studies.

Wilsnack, R. W., Vogeltanz, N. D., Wilsnack, S. C., Harris, T. R. (2000). Gender differences in alcohol consumption and adverse drinking consequences: Cross-cultural patterns. *Addiction*, **95**, 251-265.

Wilsnack, S. C., Wilsnack, R. W. (1990). Women and substance abuse: research directions for the 1990s. *Psychology of Addictive Behaviors*, **4**, 46–49.

Wilsnack, R. W., Wilsnack, S. C. (2002). International gender and alcohol research: recent findings. *Alcohol Research & Health*, **26**, 245-250.

York, J. L., Welte, J. W. (1994). Gender comparisons of alcohol consumption in alcoholic and non-alcoholic populations. *Journal of Studies on Alcohol*, **55**, 743-750.

World Health Organization (2004). *Global status report: alcohol policy*. Geneva. WHO.

Zacny, J.P. (1990). Behavioral aspects of alcohol-tobacco interactions. *Recent Developments in Alcoholism*, **8**, 205-219.

CHAPTER 4

ALCOHOL, GENDER AND PARTNER AGGRESSION: A STUDY IN THE GREATER METROPOLITAN AREA OF COSTA RICA

JULIO BEJARANO-OROZCO

INTRODUCTION

BACKGROUND

The Republic of Costa Rica is located in Central America, with Nicaragua on the north and Panama on the south, and coasts on the east and west. Its land area of 51 thousand square kilometers is comparable with the size of Switzerland. According to data from the 2000 national census (Instituto Nacional de Estadística y Censos, 2001) there are 4 million inhabitants, including nearly 14% inmigrants, especially from Nicaragua. Migrant flow occurs in response to several factors: natural disasters, political conflict and structural economic imbalances.

A Human Development Index (HDI) of 0.821 places the country in an advantageous position according to the United Nations Development Programme. Literacy rate is 96% and life expectancy for women is 80.29 years, and 76 years for men. The general mortality rate in 2002 was 3.71 per one thousand and the infant mortality rate is 11.15 children per one thousand live births. Among primary causes of death are circulatory diseases, tumors and reproductive system diseases. The prevalence of HIV infection in women aged 15-24 is 0.3%

The mortality rate with regard to alcohol-related problems in 2002 (liver disease, cirrhosis, alcoholic hepatitis, etc.) is 11.59 per one thousand deaths. The male rate is 17.23, the female rate is 3.93. From all car accidents in year 2002, one out of four involved the driver's or pedestrian's intoxication.

Alcohol consumption and alcohol-related problems have been a long-standing public health problem in Costa Rica. Alcohol-related matters have undergone change according to different historical, social and economic circumstances. One of the most important is the transformation in family functioning and in men's and women's social roles. On the other hand, most of the research on alcohol carried out in Costa Rica in the past 20 years has been done without a gender perspective, although it showed differences between men and women. Several studies (Bejarano & Sáenz, 2000; Bejarano, 2000; Jiménez & Bejarano, 1991), as well as a few other references in the Latin American context (Alcaráz et al., 1999; Rumbos, 2002) suggest that in the last 15 years or so, men have been drinking between 3 and 4 times the amount of alcohol consumed by women. Neither precise statistics nor reliable estimates of the male/female alcohol consumption ratio have been available until recent years. Since the early seventies research on alcohol and alcoholism (Miguez, 1985) has recognized that Costa Rican's alcohol consumption can be understood in large part as a way to facilitate social interaction.

The historical idea of the Costa Rican nation as peasants isolated in mountains has influenced individuals' perception of themselves, in addition to a social definition of males with a *machista* component that involves the repression of spontaneity and the repression of affective expression. In fact, youngsters received strong social pressure to keep the cultural model of behavior intact (Escobar, 1974). In this model, the meaning of alcohol is linked with social integration and drinking is defined as a way to facilitate social solidarity. Alcohol is seen a culturally legitimate way to relieve the anxiety produced by social interaction, and that is why the cultural modeling of young people includes alcohol for every social activity in which they get involved.

Since the seventies, different reports based on production and sales data have shown a low percapita consumption of alcohol (5 litres of absolute alcohol per year) when compared with developed countries. Nevertheless, drinking occasions, usually happening once or twice a week, are characterized by substantial amounts of alcohol intake.

Data available in Costa Rica since 1990 clearly show that men consume more frequently than women in all age groups (Sáenz, 1999; Jiménez & Bejarano, 1991). Men who are 20-49 years of age consume more frequently than younger and older men. According to the 1995 national survey on alcohol and drug abuse (Bejarano & San Lee, 1997), the prevalence of heavy drinking (5 or more drinks consumed per occasion) is higher in men (33.7%) than among women, whose prevalence is rather low (6%). Although there is strong evidence that male and female drinking behaviour are different, women's patterns of consumption have changed in the last 25 years (Bejarano, San Lee & Carvajal, 1999). From initial patterns of moderate consumption, women's heavy drinking levels have increased in a significant way.

Recent research from the beginning of the new century (Bejarano & Ugalde, 2003) has shown that more educated women show a higher prevalence of heavy drinking (by 10%), and research on 7th to 9th grade students suggests an earlier age of onset. In fact, the age of onset of alcohol use for both young men and women is as low as eleven years, which is lower than the age of onset found in other Latin American and even European countries (Jernigan, 2001). One main aspect with regard to the age of onset and some drinking patterns, like drunkenness, type of drinking context, etc., is the absence of gender-related significant differences. This is a matter of growing concern at the national level, and particularly true in the school-based context as compared to the general population.

The role of education, which shows special relations with drinking in different countries, the role of religion, the availability of alcohol, including its price, the role of having work and some mood-related reasons are key aspects to be surveyed in future investigations.

Costa Rica is part of the GENACIS study, a multinational study of gender, alcohol and culture, and the present work explores the relationship among individual-level and societal variables and alcohol consumption and alcohol problems in both men and women. The main variables are familial and other social settings for alcohol consumption, intimate relations and sexuality, social networks, aggression and childhood abuse, health and lifestyle, work experience, social role, gender inequality, and aspects of the drinking culture.

The objectives of the Genacis study include the following:

- Comparisons of the drinking patterns between men and women.
- Comparisons of the prevalence of alcohol-related problems between men and women.
- Comparisons of correlates of women's and men's heavy alcohol consumption and alcohol-related problems.
- Societal-level analyses of the associations between women's and men's drinking behaviour and types of drinking cultures and gender inequality.
- Development of improved culture- and gender-sensitive measures of alcohol consumption and alcohol-related problems.

This work also explores the relationship of violence/victimization and alcohol consumption in the Greater Metropolitan Area of Costa Rica, an issue which is a key topic for the Genacis project. Domestic violence in Costa Rica has a growing importance, especially violence among intimate partners, and it is recognized as a public health problem and a citizenship security issue. As pointed out by Graham, Wells and Jelley (2002), research has found higher rates of domestic violence among intimate partners who drink heavily. The connections between alcohol consumption and violence suggest that the effects of alcohol could play a causal role in aggression or increase the incidence and severity of male violence against their partners. However, there is a considerable debate about the nature of the relationship between alcohol consumption and violence, and whether it is truly causal. Some authors believe that alcohol works as a factor increasing the likelihood of aggressive behaviour or violence by reducing inhibitions, affecting judgment and impairing the ability of the drinker to interpret cues. Other authors argue that the connection between alcohol intake and violence is culturally dependent, and happens only in places where social expectancies are that drinking evokes or excuses certain behaviours (World Health Organization, 2002).

In Costa Rica partner violence accounts for a growing number of deaths of women by murder and a significant number of physical and psychological injuries. In the year 2000, the National Institute on Women (Barahona, 2002) counted four thousand cases; 36% of these were new ones, and 26% requested protection measures (e.g. requiring the partner to stay away from home).

This study explores some relevant aspects regarding alcohol consumption by males and females from the Costa Rican Greater Metropolitan Area sample, and makes a first approach to the problem of domestic violence and its relation with drinking behaviour.

METHOD

SAMPLING DESIGN

The master sample framework was obtained from the National Institute on Statistics and Census (Instituto Nacional de Estadística y Censos, INEC), and some variables were used as controlling variables, for establishing differences within groups. These were gender, age, occupation and economic condition. The sample was drawn from the Greater Metropolintan Area, a geographical area which contains almost one half of the national population and households.

The design of the study was a household survey restricted to the Greater Metropolitan Area population. It was a multistage cluster sample design including males and females aged 18 and older, living permanently or temporarily in houses. The primary sampling unit was the segment (geographical area with an arbitrary delimitation: i.e. streets, houses, rivers, including approximately 70 households), which was selected by proportional size probability, based on the number of existing households in it. The second sampling stage is the household, which was selected systematically from an initial random start. For each segment the interviewer had a detailed map to select the starting dwelling and the direction to follow. The final sample stage was the subject in each household. The subjects were selected randomly using a route sheet (i.e., a fieldwork interview selection blueprint — a document containing information about household residents for making a systematic selection of individuals).

Sample size was 1274 respondents (630 men and 644 women). Eighty-two percent of the sample was from the urban zone and 18% from rural areas. In the urban area 51.6% were men and 48.4% women, while in the rural area 39.7% were men and 60.3% women. Each face-to-face interview was made by one of eight experienced and trained advanced psychology students, administering the standardized 30-45 minute Genacis interview. Respondents were informed that they could refuse to answer any of the items of the questionnaire that they did not want to answer. Fieldworkers were also prepared to deal with any special situations regarding respondent feelings evoked by some sensitive questions (sexuality, victimization, alcohol consumption, etc.).

The sample design did not include homeless people, patients in hospitals or those without established residence. The post-hoc weighting variables were sex, age, working status and province.

MEASURES

The GENACIS questionnaire assessed demographic characteristics (e.g. gender, date of birth, family income, nationality and ethnicity, marital status, educational level), social network (informal and supportive contacts with family and non-family members), drinking patterns (drinking frequency, beverage preference, amounts of alcohol per drinking session, time spent drinking, age at onset, drinking contexts), drinking consequences, intimate relations and sexuality, violence and victimization, health and lifestyle. The response rate in this study was 96%.

Most of the quantity and frequency of drinking questions were asked for the past 12 months. Frequency responses were analyzed in terms of three main categories: more often than weekly, 1 to 3 times monthly and less than monthly. *Current drinker* is a respondent who reported consumption of any alcoholic beverage in the last 12 months. A heavy drinker is defined as a respondent who drinks five or more drinks per occasion. Lifetime abstainers are those who have never used alcohol, and current abstainers are those who had nothing to drink (including lifetime abstainers) in the twelve months preceding the interview.

Alcohol-related problems were assessed with two screening questionnaires, CAGE and AUDIT. Regarding the Audit, the hazardous alcohol use (questions 1 to 3) cut-off point was 6. The dependence (questions 4 to 6) cut-off was 4 and the harmful use (questions 7 to 10) cut-off was 7 points. The cut-off point for the whole Audit was 8+ points, which is the score that produces the highest sensitivity (Babor et al., 1992). There was also a set of questions related to drinking consequences at the individual, family and social level.

A typology of drinkers was created based on drinking amounts and the frequency of drinking:

- Infrequent light drinker: drinks less than five drinks, less than weekly;
- Frequent light drinker: drinks less than five drinks, more than weekly;
- Infrequent heavy drinker: drinks five or more drinks, less than weekly;
- Frequent heavy drinker: drinks five or more drinks, more than weekly.

For analysis purposes some other typologies were created: current abstainers vs. current drinkers; non-heavy drinkers vs. heavy drinkers; lifetime abstainers, former drinkers and current drinkers.

STATISTICAL ANALYSIS

A non-parametric test (*chi-square* with Yate's continuity correction) was used to test for differences between categorical variables. Multinomial logistic regression model was carried out to test the likelihood of changes in the dependent variable due to selected independent variables.

RESULTS

DEMOGRAPHIC CHARACTERISTICS

As shown in Table 1, the ratio of males to females in the sample was 0.98:1. Both men and women were distributed evenly, but men were more likely to be single, work in the services sector and live in an urban area. Males were also more likely than females to report a middle family income and to provide more than half of the family income.

The distribution of age groups was similar among males and females, and it also resembled the distribution at the national level. As showed by other studies (Proyecto Estado de la Nación, 2002), women's educational level was slightly higher than men's, and they also had a lower rate of unemployment and retirement status than men.

Both men and women were Catholics (not in Table) in similar proportion (almost 70%), but there was a significantly higher percentage of women having a Protestant preference (23.3% vs. 17% in males).

THE CONTEXT WHERE SPOUSES/PARTNERS LIVE

Fifty six percent of men and women were married or lived with a partner. The partners for 14% of males and 3% of females were individuals of the same sex. The average number of people living in households where the respondent was living with a partner was 4.5. About 16% of single people had ever lived with a partner. Altogether, 65% of men and 80% of women have had children (average per respondent: 2 children).

Twenty percent of men who were married or living together and 26% of women in the same condition reported an "extremely unhappy", "unhappy" or "fairly unhappy" relationship. One third of them reported that talking about feelings or problems with the partner was "very difficult", "difficult" or "fairly difficult". Fifteen percent of men reported quarreling with a partner at least several times a month, while 24% of women did the same. Just 1% of males reported the spouse/partner was drinking (at least occasionally) while quarreling compared with 12% of females reporting the spouse/partner drinking occasionally or more frequently in this circumstance. One out of four men and one out of three women have felt lonely from time to time (13% of men, 18% of women) or often and very often (13% of males, 15% of females) during the last 12 months.

For almost one third of males married or living together, over their lifetime sexuality has been *somewhat important* (23%) to *not important* (5%); 45% of women responded that way (*somewhat important:* 29% and

TABLE 1. Sociodemographic characteristics of the sample, by gender
(Weighted cases)

Variables	Male		Female	
	n	%	n	%
Age				
18-29 years	212	33.7	209	32.5
30-44 years	194	30.8	217	33.7
45+ years	224	35.5	218	33.9
Total	630	100	644	100
Marital status				
Married	249	39.5	302	46.9
Single	231	36.7	155	24.1
Living with a partner	101	16.0	87	13.4
Divorced	24	3.8	34	5.3
Widowed	14	2.3	37	5.7
Married but separated	11	1.8	29	4.6
Total	630	100	644	100
Educational level				
0-6 years	263	41.7	273	42.4
7-9 years	102	16.2	114	17.8
10-12 years	36	5.6	37	5.8
High school diploma	126	19.9	99	15.4
Bachelor's degree	59	9.4	73	11.3
Postgraduate	41	6.6	46	7.1
Don't know/Does not apply	3	0.5	1	0.2
Total	630	100	644	100
Occupation				
Services sector	194	30.9	89	13.8
Homemaker	24	3.7	379	58.8
Technician	97	15.5	38	5.9
Unemployed	81	12.9	8	1.2
Student	85	13.6	57	8.8
Professional	60	9.6	54	8.4
Retired	45	7.1	13	2.1
Agriculture	41	6.5	5	0.8
Don't know/Does not apply	3	0.3	1	0.2
Total	630	100	644	100
Income				
Low	222	35.2	293	45.7
Middle	357	56.7	299	46.5
High	47	7.5	33	5.2
Don't know/Does not apply	4	0.6	17	2.6
Total	630	100	642	100
Residence				
Urban	539	85.5	506	78.5
Rural	91	14.4	138	21.4

not important: 16%). Eight percent of males and 4% of women have had two sexual partners or more during the last twelve months.

DRINKING STATUS

There were 424 drinkers (67%) and 204 non-drinkers (lifetime abstainers and current abstainers) in the sample of 630 men, and 273 drinkers (42%) and 369 non-drinkers (57%) in the female sample of 644. The percentage of people that reported never having had any drink in their life was only 8.6% for men and 18.9% for women. This women's abstention rate is low if it is compared with countries like Mexico, where abstention percentages are considerably higher (Medina-Mora et al., 2001).

Most drinkers were in the 18-29 age group, among both men and women. Former drinkers were in the group aged 45 and older. For men and women, lifetime abstention rates decreased as education level rises. Forty percent of men and 70% of women with less than 6 years of education were lifetime abstainers or current abstainers, while this was only true for 17% of males and 57% of females that had attended school for 10 to 12 years ($p<0.005$).

The probability of being a current drinker was higher if the person had 13 years of education or more ($p<0.0001$). Among women, last year abstainers were more frequent in the low income category, and the rate of abstention decreased as the income rose ($p<0.0001$). Women were more likely than men to be abstainers ($p<0.009$) in both the urban and rural areas.

DRINKING FREQUENCY

In males, heavy drinking (drinking 5+ drinks at least once a month) was associated with the frequency of drinking ($p<0.002$), as shown on Table 2. Two thirds of males who reported frequent drinking could be

TABLE 2. **Drinking frequency by prevalence of heavy drinking and gender among current drinkers**
(weighted cases)

Drinking frequency	Men *		Women **	
	Heavy drinker (%)	n	Heavy drinker (%)	n
Weekly +	66.7	90	28.0	25
1-3 monthly	42.1	76	29.6	54
Less than monthly	47.3	258	25.8	194

* *p<0.002*
** *ns*

considered heavy drinkers, using the definition of heavy drinking as consuming at least five drinks, more than once a month. This relation was not true for women: rates of heavy drinking did not vary by frequency of drinking. This difference could be partially explained in terms of the role that culture assigns to male and female drinking.

All those men and women who drank frequently (weekly or more) preferred to drink at a bar or at home. It is interesting that males were more likely than females to drink at their workplace. Most of the respondents drink primarily on weekend evenings, according to the cultural tendency weekend episodes of alcohol intake instead of daily consumption (Table 3).

TABLE 3.   Drinking contexts, by gender and drinking frequency
(weighted cases)

Drinking context (time and day)	Drinking frequency (%)							
	Men				Women			
	weekly+	1-3 monthly	< monthly	n	weekly+	1-3 monthly	< monthly	n
Daytime, weekday	18.3	7.3	74.4	120	13.2	12.4	74.4	31
Evening, weekday	20.2	17.4	62.4	253	15.4	14.9	69.8	97
Daytime, weekend	17.1	13.7	69.2	227	7.3	17.8	74.9	92
Evening, weekend	33.3	26.6	40.1	350	15.7	21.1	63.2	243
About to drive a car	14.1	8.4	77.5	94	9.6	3.2	87.3	19

Drinking during a meal or at a party was more prevalent in those men and women who drank less than monthly, compared with those who drank weekly+ ($p<0.012$). In general, drinking at their own homes was preferred for both men and women to drinking in other places ($p<0.012$), and most of those who had low drinking frequencies preferred to drink with a family member.

HEAVY DRINKING

In the whole male sample, 34% were heavy drinkers. One out of three was a frequent heavy drinker. Among females, 11.2% were heavy drinkers and just one out of ten was a frequent heavy drinker. Among current drinkers, 50% of males and 26.6% of females drink excessively (five or more drinks per occasion).

Almost 47% of males in the 18-29 age group were either infrequent or frequent heavy drinkers, while this was true of just 20% of women in the same age group (Table 4). For both men and women, the probability of drinking heavily decreases with increasing age ($p<0.0001$).

TABLE 4.   Typology of drinking, by gender and age
(Weighted cases)

Gender	Age	Typology of drinking (%)					n
		Current Abstainer	Infrequent light	Frequent light	Infrequent heavy	Frequent heavy	
Male *	18-29	22.6	25.9	4.2	36.3	10.5	212
	30-44	29.9	34.5	3.1	17.5	14.9	194
	45+	45.1	25.9	6.7	19.2	3.1	224
Female *	18-29	48.8	29.2	2.4	18.2	1.4	209
	30-44	56.4	29.4	2.8	10.1	1.4	218
	45+	67.0	26.6	3.2	2.8	0.5	218

* $p<0.0001$

It is also interesting that men and women who have never been married are more likely to be frequent or infrequent heavy drinkers than any other marital condition ($p<0.0001$ and $p<0.012$, respectively)

DRINKING-RELATED PROBLEMS

Compared with females, male drinkers had higher rates of drinking problems. In fact, females reporting alcohol-related problems were rare. Fifteen percent of male current drinkers reported consequences for their physical health, on marriage or intimate relations, 23% reported fights while drinking, and 20% reported that their drinking affected their finances. In males, high quantity drinkers reported more alcohol-related problems than low quantity drinkers.

Using the CAGE questionnaire scores of 2 or more positive answers, drinking problems were found in 21% of current drinkers among men, and 8.7% among women. This was especially true for heavy drinkers.

One hundred and four men and 17 women had AUDIT scores of 8 or higher. These values represent 24.6% of male and 6.2% of female current drinkers. Hazardous use was present in one out of four males and in 6% of females. Among those married and living together, the rate was 20% of males and 4% of females. Harmful use existed in less than 3% of males and females.

Among males, most of those reporting any specific problem from drinking (Table 5) were heavy drinkers, whether the problem was with

TABLE 5. Drinking related problems: proportion of each attributable to non-heavy and heavy drinkers, by gender
(Weighted cases)

Drinking related problem	Men			Women		
	Non-heavy drinkers (%)	Heavy drinkers (%)	n	Non-heavy drinkers (%)	Heavy drinkers (%)	n
On work, studies or employment opportunities	9.1	90.9	33 *	0	100	5 *
On housework or chores around the house	10.0	90.0	20 *	33.3	66.7	9 **
On marriage/intimate relationships	9.4	90.6	64 *	20.0	80.0	5 **
On relationships with other family members	6.1	93.9	49 *	38.9	61.1	18 ***
On friendships or social life	4.0	96.0	25 *	33.3	66.7	6 ***
On physical health	19.0	81.0	63 *	40.0	60.0	25 *
On finances	16.5	83.5	85 *	13.3	86.7	15 *
Got in trouble with the law	23.1	76.9	26 **	0	100	1
Got an illness connected with drinking	26.7	73.3	15	80.0	20.0	5
Lost a job, or nearly lost one	21.4	78.6	28 ***	100	0	1
Annoyed by people criticizing drinking	18.3	81.7	82 *	39.3	60.7	28 *
Spouse or partner threatened to leave or left	19.4	80.6	36 *	66.7	33.3	6
Lost a friendship because of the drinking	27.3	72.7	11	33.3	66.7	3
Gotten in a fight while drinking	19.2	88.8	99 *	35.3	64.7	17 ***

* p<0.0001
** p<0.005
***p<0.002
Note: Caution is called for when sample size is lower than 20 cases.

work, with relationships, with physical health, or in terms of getting into a fight. Among women reporting specific problems, the predominance of heavy drinkers was generally less, with other drinkers accounting for up to 40% of those reporting problems with physical health, with relationships with family members, and in terms of getting into a fight after drinking.

VIOLENCE AND VICTIMIZATION

Heavy drinkers were more likely to have been pushed, punched, grabbed, slapped or threatened than non-heavy drinkers (p<0.05). This was the case both for female and for male current drinkers ($p<0.0001$).

Physically aggressive things were more likely to have happened to divorced, separated or widowed males ($p<0.0001$) than to those in any other marital condition (Table 6). It is possible that there exists a relationship between the condition of being a divorced or separated male and the aggressive act reported. This relationship was not found among females.

TABLE 6. **Aggressive things done to repondents, by gender and marital status**
(weighted cases)

Gender	Marital status	The most physically aggressive thing done to respondent				
		None (%)	Push, punch, kick, grab, slap (%)	Threaten /threaten with weapon (%)	n	*p value*
Male	Married/living together	95.1	2.9	2.0	350	
	Divorced, widowed, separated	83.7	2.0	14.3	49	0.0001
	Never married	85.7	12.6	1.7	231	
Female	Married/living together	89.2	8.2	2.6	388	
	Divorced, widowed, separated	91.1	6.9	2.0	101	0.165
	Never married	95.5	4.5	0	153	

Among males and females married or living together, those scoring 8+ in the AUDIT were more likely to be victims of physical aggression than those whose scores were lower ($p<0.003$). Also males scoring 8+ were more likely than those with lower scores to do physically aggressive things to their intimate partners ($p<0.0001$).

It is interesting that rates of partner aggression (both the most physically aggressive thing done to the respondent and the most physically aggressive things done to others by the respondent during the last 2 years) were similar in men and women in the whole sample. In fact 9% of males and 9.2% of females reported physically aggressive things done to them, as well as 5% reporting physically aggressive things done by them. The first finding has also been shown by various studies (Archer, 2000). But it does not necessarily mean that the levels of male and female aggression involved were the same. Graham et al. (2002) have pointed out that although rates of partner aggression are similar for both genders, the dynamics and the role of alcohol are gender-specific. Among people married or living together, there are more females than males reporting that they have been subjects of aggression ($p<0.0001$). In women, living with someone now or in the past increases the probability of suffering physically aggressive acts. This finding is supported by studies which have shown that a woman who lives with a heavy drinker has a greater risk of physical violence from her partner (World Health Organization, 2002).

It is clear then that aggressive actions are more likely between males and females if they are heavy drinkers ($p<0.0001$). Aggressive actions were also more present in low income males ($p<0.0001$) than in those with middle or high income. The probability of occurrence of these physically aggressive actions was higher if respondents were current drinkers ($p<0.009$ in men, $p<0.005$ in women), if they started to drink at age 13 years or less ($p<0,002$), and if their current age was 30-34 years ($p<0.012$).

Considering the most physically aggressive thing in the last two years done to males, 17% of the respondents had been drinking before the event, while 15.3% of the perpetrators had been drinking ($p<0.050$). Seventy five percent of males and females indicated that it was the spouse/partner who had perpetrated the aggressive actions, and for more than a half of male respondents the action happened once. Two thirds of males reported that the intensity of this act was low. Just one third of women said the same. Interestingly, evidence from elsewhere (World Health Organization, 2002) indicates that men who have been drinking prior to a violent act inflict more serious violence at the time of the aggressive event.

Regarding the most physically aggressive act committed by the respondent (Table 7), one third of males reported alcohol consumption before the event, while just 7.5% of females were drinking ($p<0.020$). The intensity of the action was low, according to 83% of males and 68.5% of females. The spouse/partner was the victim, according to 84.4% of males and 69.2% of females. Concerning the emotional impact of violence,

TABLE 7. **Aggressive things done by the respondent, by gender and type of drinker**
(weighted cases)

Gender	Type of drinker	The most physically aggressive thing done by respondent			n	p value
		None (%)	Push, punch, kick, grab, slap (%)	Threaten /threaten with weapon (%)		
Male	Not heavy drinker	98.8	1.2	0	416	0.0001
	Heavy drinker	87.4	11.7	0.9	214	
Female	Not heavy drinker	95.3	4.4	0.4	570	0.007
	Heavy drinker	86.1	12.5	1.4	72	

Graham et al. (2002) argue that there are gender differences, with men experiencing less emotional impact than women from events of physical violence.

The number of times in the last 12 months that males and females were insulted or sworn at was related to being a heavy drinker ($p<0.012$).

In general, results of this study are consistent with findings reported in the social science literature on risk factors for physically assaulting an intimate partner. For example, Black et al. (1999) have indicated that among demographic factors, being younger and having a low income were consistently found to be factors associated with the likelihood of a man committing physical violence against a partner. Heavy drinking appears to be a risk factor for partner violence.

Two different multinomial logistic regression models were created to test the association between physical aggression and selected predictor variables. The dependent variable used in the models corresponded to either being the perpetrator of aggressive acts on an intimate partner (Table 8) or being the victim of aggressive acts (Table 9). Each of the two variables was recoded as "Did and did not commit or experience any aggressive act".

The models contained all those individuals who drank in the past year (current drinkers). The following were independent variables used in this analysis:

- Gender (male, female);
- Age group (18-29; 30-44 and 45+);

- Intimate partner's number of drinks in a typical day (reported by respondent);

- Type of drinker (infrequent light, frequent light, infrequent heavier and frequent heavier);

- Intimate partner's drinking frequency (every day or nearly every day, three or four times a week, once or twice a week, one to three times a month, seven to eleven times in the last 12 months, three to six times in the last 12 months, twice in the last 12 months, once in the last 12 months);

- AUDIT score (recoded as 0 to 7 and 8+);

- Methods to solve disagreements (almost without quarreling, sometimes having short-lived quarrels or disagreements, often having long-lasting quarrels for different reasons, not only quarrel but having physical fights).

It was not possible to build the model controlling for drinking or not drinking before the aggressive incident due to the small number of observations (less than 15 cases).

For every model, it was necessary to observe the Goodness of Fit test, which indicates the feasibility to continue or not with the construction of the model, and the Chi Square test for the dependent variable, which is used to check the null hypothesis that the sample came from a population in which data occurred with a specific probability. To identify regression coefficients that were significantly different from zero, the Wald-Wolfowitz non-parametric test was used. This tests the hypothesis that two samples come from the same population; if the samples come from the same population, both groups should scatter randomly through sorted data.

TABLE 8. **Multinomial logistic regression model predicting aggression to intimate partner (current drinkers only)**

Variables	Exp (B)	95% CI for Exp(B)	
		Lower limit	*Upper limit*
Gender	0.8625	0.2280	3,2624
Age group	0.5163	0.2252	1.1834
Number of drinks drunk by respondent	1.0678	0.9296	1.2265
Type of drinker (respondent)	1.3329	0.6931	2.5637
Intimate partner's drinking frequency	1.1647	0.7006	1.3962
Intimate partner's number of drinks drunk	1.3713	1.9654	1.4049
Respondent's AUDIT score	1.7964	0.4703	6.8623
Method of disagreement resolution	0.6017	0.2757	1.3128

N = 191; CI = confidence interval
Chi-Square for the model = 21.930 with 7 DF, (p<0.005)

TABLE 9. **Multinomial logistic regression model predicting aggression to respondent (current drinkers only)**

Variables	Exp (B)	95% CI for Exp(B)	
		Lower limit	*Upper limit*
Gender	0.0859	0.0190	0.3883
Age group	0.5117	0.2355	1.1115
Number of drinks drunk by respondent	0.9692	0.8253	1.1382
Type of drinker (intimate partner)	0.7773	0.3924	1.5396
Intimate partner's drinking frequency	1.4251	0.9492	2.1394
Intimate partner's number of drinks drunk	1.3713	1.1034	1.7043
Respondent's AUDIT score	1.1275	0.2549	4.9881
Method of disagreement resolution	0.7773	0.6495	2.5481

N = 191; CI = confidence interval
Chi-Square for the model = 72.191 with 7 DF, (p<0.0001)

There were no statistically significant coefficients. Nevertheless, age and amount of drinks drunk by the repondent in a typical day showed some type of association with the commission of a physically aggressive act (Table 8). In the model built from the dependent variable "the most physically aggressive thing done to the respondent," significant coefficients included gender, age, intimate partner's drinking frequency, and intimate partner's amount of drinks consumed in a typical day (Table 9). Being female and young were significantly associated with the experiences of physical violence, and partner's drinking frequency and amount of consumption were positively related to violence. Gender was the predictor with the strongest association with the dependent variable.

Partner's number of drinks was related to violence in a direct way. The regression analyses suggest that when the respondent was the object of aggression it was more likely that his/her alcohol use (type of drinker, AUDIT score, drinking frequency and amount of drinks consumed) affected the dependent measure.

DISCUSSION AND CONCLUSIONS

This study shows that rates of abstention in both the urban and the rural population are quite low. In fact, being a current drinker is prevalent in most of the population and especially in younger men and women.

The patterns of alcohol consumption are affected by educational level. Although drinking correlates positively with the level of education in both men and women, this relationship could not be established for heavy drinking, where education seems to play a different role and where other variables may have a stronger influence. The relation of heavy drinking with such variables as having never been married and being in younger age groups suggests that these segments deserve close surveillance in terms of prevention. Certainly, females drink less frequently and their rates of heavy drinking are lower than men, but this study also shows that levels of drinking and heavy drinking are rising if the situation is compared with survey data from the 1980s and the 1990s, at least in the Greater Metropolitan Area.

Results from this study suggest that heavy drinking is linked with a significant risk of alcohol-related problems, a fact which indicates that attention should be paid more to the hazardous use of alcohol than to abstaining versus drinking. Hazardous use of alcohol implies a high risk of damage to health, even if this risk has not yet resulted in significant physical or mental ill effects. This reinforces the idea of addressing acute intoxication as a goal of problem prevention. Ours is a culture which promotes heavy drinking among specific groups of the population and does not limit drinking, as occurs in cultures with traditions of temperate drinking. Policymakers should attend to the problem of drinking large amounts of alcohol at one sitting, linked to specific risks, which calls for promotion of drinking moderation and public education on the risks involved in drinking large quantities of alcohol in short periods of time.

A rapid increase in alcohol intake would raise the probability of further increases in alcohol-related problems in coming years. This is especially true if patterns of consumption of teenagers still within the educational system, which at this point are considered critical, are taken into account.

This study also reveals that alcohol is a risk marker for partner violence. In fact, the data show that alcohol abuse and even just alcohol intake are related to violence. Although men and women reported similar rates of aggression by partners, women reported greater fear and severity of aggression. For preventive purposes, it would be important to consider the link between alcohol consumption, a low income situation and younger age status as factors which increase the risk of violence in men.

In Costa Rica, where women's status is clearly in transition (in terms of their educational level, the fact of working out of home and being the family head, new legislation protecting them against domestic and work violence and promoting equalities, the gender perspective within the educational system, etc.), it could be hypothesized that the risk of violence from intimate partners is higher. However, this relationship and the possibility that high status women have a lower risk of violence should be studied carefully.

Public concern with alcohol-related problems is not new in Costa Rica. Different and isolated efforts have been carried out since the beginning of the previous century, but it was not until the early 1990s that resources and activities were integrated within a nationwide plan. This still needs to be converted into a national policy that integrates not only the need for treatment of chronic cases but health promotion and specific and non-specific prevention in the educational system, as well as measures targeting alcohol availability, taxation policies, advertising regulations, legal enforcement of underage drinking and intoxication in public places. All these issues should be considered under the thesis that drinking patterns are better predictors of negative and positive consequences than solely the idea of per capita consumption. And that is why it is also necessary to consider at the national level the practice of harm reduction instead of promoting abstinence per se. A harm reduction approach would promote those drinking patterns that maximize individual health and quality of life and improve the measures leading to reductions of the risk and severity of adverse consequences arising from alcohol consumption. However, it is important to determine which drinking patterns are harmful and which ones are not and how information on this can be disseminated widely.

National concern about domestic violence is more recent and the link between alcohol and violence is emerging as a matter of public discussion. In terms of violence and victimization issues, it is important to point out that how a community responds to partner violence may affect the overall levels of abuse in the community. Finally, it is important to suggest that governments should invest much more in research on violence by intimate partners.

ACKNOWLEDGEMENTS

This work was possible because of the participation of many people. First, the statistician Oscar Acuña helped in performing the statistical analysis, especially the multinomial logistic regression models. Andrea Cuenca was the fieldwork leader and coordinated the work of Maribel Calderon, Ivon Gutierrez, Carolina Gutierrez, Sebastián Alfaro, Karla Leiva, Manuel Coto, Andrea Brenes and Giselle Amador. Leda Vargas assisted in administrative support from the Fundación Vida y Sociedad.

REFERENCES

Alcaráz, F. et al. (1999). El consumo de drogas en Bolivia (Drug use in Bolivia). La Paz, Bolivia: CELIN.

Archer, J. (2000). Sex differences in aggression between heterosexual partners: a meta-analytic review. *Psychological Bulletin*, **126**, 651-680.

Barahona, V. (2002). La violencia doméstica y su relación con el consumo de sustancias psicoactivas en la mujer: un estudio realizado en la Delegación de la Mujer de San José (Domestic violence and its relationship with women's drug use: a study made at the Woman's Delegation of San José). (Tesis SEP). San José, C.R.: UCR.

Babor, T et al. (1992) AUDIT: the Alcohol Use Disorders Identification Test: Guidelines for use in Primary Health Care. Geneva: WHO/PSA/92.4.

Black, DA, et al. (1999) Partner, child abuse risk factor literature review: National Network of Family Resiliency. National Network for Health (online) Available at: http://www.nnh.org/risk

Bejarano, J., Ugalde, F. (2003). Consumo de drogas en Costa Rica. Resultados de la Encuesta Nacional del 2000-2001 (Drug use in Costa Rica. Outcomes from the National Household Survey, 2000/2001). San José, Costa Rica: I.A.F.A

Bejarano, J., Sáenz, M. (2000). Consumo de drogas y muerte violenta en Costa Rica (Drug use and violent death in Costa Rica). *Adicciones*, **12**(3), 435-441.

Bejarano, J. (2000). Alcohol Epidemiology in Costa Rica. In: Demers, A., Room, R. & Bougault, C.. Eds. *Surveys of Drinking Patterns and Problems in Seven Developing Countries*. Geneva: World Health Organization, pp. 33-44.

Bejarano, J., San Lee, L. (1997). Alcohol y alcoholismo en la sociedad Costarricense (Alcohol and alcoholism in Costarican society). *Revista de Ciencias Sociales*, **77**, 9-20.

Bejarano, J., San Lee, L. & Carvajal, H. (1999). El consumo de drogas en la mujer costarricense (Drug use among Costa Rican women). *Revista de Ciencias Sociales*, **22**(2), 41-48.

Escobar, F. (1974). San Ramón. Un estudio antropológico (San Ramón. An anthropologic study). Centro de Estudios sobre Alcoholismo, San José, C.R.

Graham, K., Wells, S. & Jelley, J. (2002). The social context of physical aggression among adults. *The Journal of Interpersonal Violence*, **17**(1), 64-83.

Graham, K. et al. (2002). Alcohol, gender and partner aggression: a general population study of adults, Ontario, Canada: Centre for Addiction and Mental Health. (in press).

Instituto Nacional de Estadística y Censos (2001). IX Censo Nacional de Población y V de Vivienda del 2000: Resultados Generales (IX National census on Population and V household census, 2000: General results), San José, C.R.: INEC

Jernigan, D. (2001). *Global Status Report: Alcohol and young people*. Geneva: World Health Organization.

Jiménez, F., & Bejarano, J. (1991). Estudio nacional sobre consumo de alcohol y drogas ilícitas (National household survey on alcohol and illicit drug consumption), San José, C.R.: IAFA.

Medina-Mora, M. et al. (2001). Patterns of alcohol consumption and related problems in Mexico: results from two general population surveys. In: Demers, A., Room, R. And Bourgault, Ch. eds. *Surveys of drinking patterns and problems in seven developing countries*. Geneva: World Health Organization, (pp. 14-31).

Miguez, H. (1985). Epidemiología de la farmacodependencia juvenil (Epidemiology of youthful drug dependence). *Boletín del Instituto Interamericano del Niño*, **223**:23-30.

Proyecto Estado de la Nación (2003). Estado de la nación en desarrollo humano sostenible (Project on Nation's Human Development), 1ª. Edición, Litografía e imprenta Lil, S.A.

Rumbos (2002). Juventud y consumo de sustancias psicoactivas (Youth and psycoactive drug use), Bogotá, COL: Arte Laser Pub. Ltda.

Sáenz, M. (1999). La prohibición de la publicidad de las bebidas alcohólicas: una prioridad en el sector salud (The ban of alcohol advertising: a priority of health sector). *Revista de Trabajo Social*, **55**, 1154-1162.

World Health Organization (2002). *World report on violence and health*. Geneva: World Health Organization.

CHAPTER 5

WOMEN AND ALCOHOL USE IN INDIA

VIVEK BENEGAL, MADHABIKA NAYAK, PRATIMA MURTHY, PRABHA CHANDRA &
G. GURURAJ

XI: 13. Drinking (spirituous liquor), associating with wicked people, separation from the husband, rambling abroad, sleeping (at unseasonable hours), and dwelling in other men's houses, are the six causes of the ruin of women.

XI: 80. A wife who drinks spirituous liquor, is of bad conduct, rebellious, diseased, mischievous, or wasteful, may at any time be superseded (by another wife).

- The Laws of Manu c. 200 A.D.

INTRODUCTION

Research on drinking patterns among women generally shows that women drink less than men (Wilsnack, 1996), across the developing (Assanangkornchai et al., 2003, Wei et al., 1999) and the developed world (Kraus et al., 2000). In fact, in all countries and historical periods studied, men have consumed more alcohol and reported more alcohol-related problems than women (Fillmore et al., 1997). Reports from India on women's drinking are sparse. Whatever data exists suggests that there are extreme gender differences in the prevalence of alcohol use.

There is general agreement that alcohol use is low in the population as a whole. The National Household Survey of Drug and Alcohol Abuse 2000-01 (Ray et al., 2004), conducted on a nationally representative sample of males, estimated that 26% of male adults had ever used alcohol, while the prevalence of current users was 21.4%. Previous studies of male drinkers showed wide variations in estimates of prevalence between different regions of the country (16.7 percent in Madras city in southern India to 49.6 percent in a Punjab village in northwest India). The prevalence of alcohol use among women (wherever data is available) has consistently been estimated at less than 5 percent (Mahal, 2000; Mohan et al.,1999; Isaac, 1998; Sundaram et al., 1984).

There is also a widespread notion that alcohol use is confined to tribal women, women of lower socio-economic status, commercial sex workers and to a limited upper crust of the rich, and not favored by women from the middle or upper socioeconomic classes (Ray and Sharma, 1994; Kumar & Parthasarathy, 1994). The dominant stereotype strongly associates alcohol use with the *primitive and/or poor*, the *immoral* and the *privileged* (Rahman,2002; Musgrave & Stern, 1988, Thimmaiah, 1979). Alcohol use, in general and especially with reference to women's use, is still negatively associated with notions of virtue.

Sexist attitudes to women's drinking persist all over the world (Blume, 1997), and in most cultures there is a greater stigma attached to drinking by females than among males. In India, proscriptions against women drinking exist from ancient times, being only one among a multitude of gender discriminatory practices which have continued almost unchanged till this day. An example of this is an injunction contained in the ancient Brahminical text on personal law, the *Manusmriti* (circa 200 A.D.), which warns that *"drinking (spirituous liquor), associating with wicked people , separation from the husband, rambling abroad, sleeping (at unseasonable hours), and dwelling in other men's houses, are the six causes of the ruin of women"* (Doniger,1991).

The public discourse on alcohol in India, has traditionally focused on the plight of women at the receiving end of alcohol-related violence and impoverishment. The founding fathers of the Indian republic highlighted this aspect while debating the inclusion of the principle of prohibition as a Directive Principle of State Policy in the Indian Constitution in 1952. The media has highlighted the role of women at the forefront of anti-alcohol agitations, perpetuating the image of women as champions of temperance (Pande, 2000; Ilaiah, 1992).

This has implications for both health promotion and alcohol services. It serves to marginalize the issue of alcohol use in women, which in turn de-legitimizes help-seeking for alcohol-related problems. Cultural attitudes in

---

Box 1: The media on women's drinking

"Economic independence, changing roles in society, entry of women into male dominated areas, economic and social emancipation, greater acceptability of social drinking and easy availability of alcohol have strongly contributed to rising incidence of alcohol consumption in women. Adolescents hit the bottle because of reasons that could range from depression to peer pressure, glamour and disappearing stereotypes about femininity."

Article in the Deccan Herald newspaper of Bangalore, July 2003

DH News Service Bangalore (2003)

"Over the last three or four years, alcohol abuse amongst women has increased...while the lower income women take to country liquor and the likes, it's the upwardly mobile yuppie women influenced as she is by a western culture, by peer pressure, by the aggressive marketing on the television, where liquor advertise-ments show gorgeous young men and women living life king-size, that finally gets to her. Sometimes, these liquor companies sponsor major events where complimentary drinks are served. Or three to four women meet together go to a pub and drink.... The young urban woman has taken to alcohol as a way of knocking down social barriers and gaining acceptance amongst her peers. Coming equipped with a strong academic, professional or family background is no longer enough. Alcohol has become the unisex leveler, an equaliser that promises instant entry amongst favoured circles. This is true of girls and women who have come from smaller towns to make a name and fortune in bigger cities".

-- Ray, S (2002). Why women get addicted to alcohol. The Tribune, April 21, Chandigarh, India.

India (being intensely guilt-provoking and discriminatory about the use of alcohol by females, though not by males) may prevent them from spontaneously reporting such details. Help-seeking is delayed until physical or psychological crises precipitate medical consultations (Murthy et al., 1995). However, there are indications that this picture may be changing. The popular media is full of accounts of increasing consumption among young women, especially in the urban setting [see Box 1].

A study of drinking habits conducted in Bangalore city (Kumar, 1997) reported that a fifth of young people who frequented pubs on weekends were girls aged between 13-19 years. Interviews with women drinkers identified boredom and lack of work at home as factors for drinking among the high-income group; the low-income group identified fatigue and spousal violence as triggers for drinking.

One of the highest rated television programmes in India is a nightly programme called *Night Out* which airs every night, after the prime-time news. This programme covers in great detail young men and women in the larger cities of the country partying at various clubs, restaurants and discotheques. Prominently featured are the regular brand launches of alcoholic beverages.

For anyone who would dismiss this as a limited urban upper class phenomenon, the reality is that India no longer lives exclusively in villages. 305 million Indians live in nearly 3700 towns and cities spread across the length and breadth of the country. This comprises 38% of its population, in sharp contrast to only 60 million (15%) who lived in urban areas in 1947 when the country became independent. At the same time, the labor force participation rate – an indication of the number of people offering themselves to be employed - came down between 1999 to 2002, for rural males (from 876 per 1000 to 858 per 1000), rural females (470 per 1000 to 423 per 1000) and urban males (796 per 1000 to 791 per 1000). However for urban females it rose in that period from 193 to 205 per 1000.

In the international literature, changes in women's education, employment, social status and economic independence have been implicated in the *convergence* of male and female drinking patterns. Neve et al. (1996) held that as women gradually acquire equal rights in work and social situations, this might also be reflected in a propensity to drink in equal amounts and in the same manner as men. While this may not explain changes in drinking patterns of non-working females, it does reflect a general change in societal attitudes to women's drinking.

The little information that exists about patterns of alcohol use in India indicate that women who do drink at all have patterns of equally heavy alcohol use as men. A study from southern India of a representative sample of 7445 adult men and 6919 adult women (Benegal et al., 2003) found that the average consumption on typical drinking occasions, in both men and women, was five standard drinks (12 gm. of ethanol per drink).

Box 2: What people drink in India

A. Reported Consumption (Legally produced alcoholic beverages)

1] Indian Made Foreign Liquor (IMFL). Refers to whisky, rum, vodka, gin and brandy with ethanol content of 42.8% by volume (75° proof). Whisky accounts for 60% of the IMFL market.

2] Country liquor (termed desi sharab in North India and arrack in South India) at 33.3 % ethanol by volume (65° proof) marketed as a standardised separate cheap low end product for the consumption of poorer sections of the population (blue collar workers in urban areas and labourers in rural areas).

> IMFL is consumed by the middle and high income groups, primarily in urban areas, however in the last decade cheap IMFL has been displacing country liquors, with a few states going so far as to ban the sales of country liquor resulting in a switch to IMFL by country liquor customers.

> The basic material in the manufacture of non-premium IMFL and of arrack is rectified spirit manufactured from molasses [e.g. Karnataka Excise Rules -Regulation of Yield, Production and Wastage of Spirit, Beer, Wine or Liquors, 1997].

3] Beer is sold as mild beer (ethanol content of 5% by volume) and strong beer (ethanol content 7.5-8%). The market is dominated by the `strong beer' brands which account for 70% of beer sales.

4] The market for wines produced in the country is miniscule but is growing at the rate of 20 to 30 per cent annually, whereas beer sales grow at 2 per cent and 3 per cent (mild and strong respectively) and IMFL figures seem to be stagnating.

5] Flavoured alcoholic beverages (FABs) appeared in the market in 2003, headed by the international brand Bacardi Breezer.

B. Unreported Consumption

Above 40% of total alcohol consumption in the country is unreported. This is mainly due to three factors.

1] The unaccounted escape of beverage alcohol, chiefly IMFL, from the legal production and supply chain, for the purpose of evading excise duties, which is then sold in the market. In popular parlance these are known as "seconds" and are usually indistinguishable from the licit variety of beverages on sale, except when they are sold cheaper than the minimum administered retail prices.

2] There is also a considerable volume of smuggling of alcoholic beverages, especially scotch whisky, into the country. With liberalization of imports this sector is becoming less important, although it still accounts for a sizeable proportion of unrecorded consumption, especially in the larger cities.

> Alcohol production, sales and its taxation are state subjects not mandated by a single federal structure. Each state has different laws governing the production, sales, duty structure and distribution. Import and export duties result in the high cost of inter-state movements, which has resulted in each state having attributes of a separate market. This naturally has proved to be an incentive for large scale smuggling of alcoholic beverages across state borders. 'Seconds' smuggled from one state into another with higher taxation are popularly called 'thirds'.

3] Illegal small scale manufacture of alcoholic beverages. A lot of it consists of traditional home-brewed beverages, which have over the years been supplanted by government-regulated industrial production and suppressed and stigmatized by the profit/revenue considerations of the liquor baron-government nexus. However, a greater proportion of this illicit brewing and distillation in relatively recent times has been taken over by small underground networks, which are often criminalized. This is especially so in rural parts, which make up over 70% of the country's population.

> Illicit liquor usually consists of a distillate of a fermented wash, comprising a variety of ingredients, like fruits and grains. Additional substances added to increase the 'kick' include rotten fruit, tree bark, molasses; copper sulphate and a small dose of methyl alcohol. Occasional additives reportedly include cowdung, chicken droppings, disused footwear, cockroaches, frogs, lizards, rats and the innards of slain fowl.

4] Low alcohol-content home-made beverages have been customarily drunk, although deemed illicit today. Toddy, the fermented sap of the coconut palm, is drunk all along the coast. Rice or millet beer is common among the tribal settlements of large sections of the country, as is the fermented drink from the mahua flower.

Licit spirits (Indian made foreign liquors, government licensed country liquor) along with illicitly distilled spirits constituted more than 95% of the beverages drunk by both men and women. Beer accounted for less than 5% of consumption (Box 2). Per capita consumption at 2 litres/adult /year (calculated from 2003 sales and population figures), after adjustment for undocumented consumption (45-50% of total consumption), is likely to be around 4 litres, but is still low compared to that in 'wet' nations. However, patterns of consumption are better indices of the likelihood of harm in the population. Repeated observations from various places in the country have documented that more than 50% of all drinkers satisfy criteria for hazardous drinking. In the study quoted previously (Benegal et al., 2003), 80% of male consumers and 65% of female consumers drank at hazardous levels (AUDIT scores of eight and above). This challenges the received wisdom that women are less likely than men to drink heavily or with adverse consequences (Plant et al., 2000; Hibell et al., 2001; Grant, 1998; Wilsnack and Wilsnack, 1997; Plant, 1997; Pittman and White, 1991).

The signature pattern is one of heavy drinking, typically more than 5 standard drinks on typical occasions. There is surprisingly little difference between amounts drunk by men and women.

A large proportion of drinkers of both genders drink daily or almost daily. Of course, the frequency is significantly higher in men. Under-socialized, solitary drinking of mainly spirits, drinking to intoxication and expectancies of drink-related disinhibition and violence add to the hazardous patterns (Gaunekar et al., 2004; Gupta et al., 2003; Benegal et al., 2003; Saxena, 1999).

Needless to say, this translates into significant alcohol-related morbidity. Alcohol-related problems account for over a fifth of hospital admissions (Sri et al., 1997, Benegal et al., 2001) but are underrecognized by primary care physicians. Alcohol misuse has been implicated in over 20% of traumatic brain injuries (Gururaj, 2002), and 60% of all injuries reporting to emergency rooms (Benegal et al., 2002). It has a disproportionately high association with deliberate self-harm (Gururaj & Isaac, 2001), high-risk sexual behavior, HIV infection (Chandra et al., 2003), tuberculosis (Rajeshwari et al., 2002), esophageal cancer (Chitra et al., 2004), liver disease and duodenal ulcer (Sarin et al., 199 ; Jain et al., 1999).

Alcohol misuse wreaks a high social cost (Bhatt, 1998; Rao et al., 2001). A study from southern India documented that monetizable direct and indirect costs attributable to alcohol, counting only persons with alcohol dependence, were more than 3 times the profits from alcohol taxation (Benegal et al., 2000). Yet, there is inadequate recognition that alcohol misuse is a major public health problem in India.

Women experience different alcohol problems than men and physical problems are experienced earlier in female drinking careers than males (Hommer et al., 2001; Holman et al., 1996; Van Thiel and Gavaler, 1988).

Three hospital-based studies of female alcoholics from southern India (Prasad et al., 1998; Murthy et al., 1995) reported patterns of solitary drinking and a high incidence of medical and psychiatric morbidity with help-seeking delayed till physical health or emotional crises made it inevitable.

While the numbers are still low, the likely conjunction of a growing consumer base of women with the prevalent motif of hazardous alcohol use will dramatically increase the public health consequences of alcohol abuse, in a country where the social cost due to alcohol in men is already alarming (Benegal et al., 2000). Regulatory measures in current use [see Box 3] are insufficiently implemented and do rather little to curb consumption.

While alcohol researchers in India, by and large, have ignored the subject of female drinkers, the alcohol industry has not. A study on the emerging beverage alcohol market in India, undertaken by the Rabobank group, clearly spells out that "the consumer base for alcohol in India will gradually expand. The target segment (men between the ages of 20 and 59), estimated to be around 23% of the Indian population, is expected to grow by 3.4% annually, to 260 million by the year 2006. Taken together with the socio-economic changes that are occurring, this makes India one of the most attractive markets for overseas investors. There are also many potential consumers to be found in other segments of the population. The introduction of new products such as flavoured and mild alcoholic products [is] aimed to recruit non-drinkers and is targeted primarily at women" (Naik, 2002).

On the face of it, there is evidence then that women's drinking is increasingly a matter of concern in India. The current study was undertaken to investigate not only the prevalence and patterns of drinking in women, but also to explore the likelihood that there are ongoing changes in the status of women's alcohol consumption in the country.

> **Box 3. Regulatory Measures in Current Use**
>
> Taxation is largely based on the volume of alcoholic beverages rather than on their strength. This encourages and promotes the use of stronger beverages as it is cheaper per unit of ethanol to buy spirits than beer or wine. Multi - point excise duties and sales taxes constitute loopholes for evasion.
>
> Existing Regulations against Sales and Retail are not effectively used:
>
> a) Prohibition of sales of alcoholic beverages to children below 18 years
>
> b) Restriction of sales at retail shops between 9 p.m. and 9 a.m.
>
> c) Prohibition of sales of alcoholic beverages in pubs, hotels etc. between 2.30 p.m. and 5.30 p.m. and after 10 p.m.
>
> d) Prohibition of setting up retail outlets within 1 km radius of schools, places of worship etc .
>
> e) Attempts to regulate the sales and consumption of alcohol along the state highways.
>
> f) Restrictions against drinking and driving or operating heavy machinery, including a Breath Alcohol Limit of 30mg %.
>
> Advertising: Although advertising of alcoholic beverages and tobacco products is banned, several companies get past this regulation by means of surrogate advertising. The norms regarding advertising of beverage alcohol are insufficiently enforced.

METHOD

The current study is part of a collaborative multi-national study (GENACIS - Gender, Alcohol, and Culture: An International Study) designed by the International Research Group on Gender and Alcohol (IRGGA), a group of researchers from more than 30 countries, affiliated with the Kettil Bruun Society for Social and Epidemiological Research on Alcohol. Using a similar methodology in a number of countries, this initiative was planned to study gender and cultural differences with regard to alcohol consumption and alcohol-related problems.

SAMPLING STRATEGY

The sheer size of India [pop. 1.03 billion – 2001 Census], and the complexity of terrain, makes a national survey difficult and costly to undertake. It was thus decided to sample an entire state (province), which would include both urban and rural areas and would be likely to have a population with varied drinking patterns, rather than being a region of abstainers only.

The state of Karnataka in southern India [pop. 52.7 million; Census of India 2001] was chosen for the study. The four southern states account for more than 25% of the national beverage alcohol market share (2000 figures) and have over the last few years experienced a significant growth rate in sales (150% in the period 1999-2000, compared to 3% in the northern sates, 58% in the eastern states, -3% in the western states and 28% overall in the country). The expectation was that this region would yield a reasonable sample of alcohol users. In view of the recent spurt in sales of alcoholic beverages, as well as the changes in women's education and employment rates noted above, it was reasonable to suppose that the convergence hypothesis could be tested within these conditions. In addition, a large epidemiological study (Benegal et al., 2003) on the prevalence of alcohol use among men and women had recently been undertaken in the southern state of Karnataka, and it was felt that re-sampling in the same region would provide both a comparison as well as a means of validating the earlier data.

Karnataka covers 192,000 square kilometers, and in many ways represents an appropriate region to undertake such research. The sex ratio of the total population of Karnataka is 1000: 964 and the corresponding figure for India is 1000:933. Average, nationally, in terms of human development indices, Karnataka also includes the urban agglomeration of Bangalore, which has been rated by the World Bank as the fastest growing city in the world and one where there has been recent socioeconomic churning. Yet in the northern districts, the state has some of the poorest and least developed areas in the country. With a population of 52 million, the state spans a variegated spectrum, and each of the four natural regions has its distinctive geographical, cultural and socioeconomic characteristics: 1] a densely populated and rich coastal region, with extensive cultivation of rice, other cash crops and with high female literacy and low child mortality; 2] a mountainous densely forested area, rich in rubber, coffee and spice plantations, similarly high on human development indices (HDI); 3] fertile riverine districts, with middling HDI and 4] the barren and arid lands in north of the state, which has one of the lowest standards of human development in the country (eight of the districts of Karnataka have female and male literacy rates below that of sub-Saharan African countries).

Five districts of the 27 in the state were identified, based on their representativeness, in that they represented the four natural regions in the state. The Bangalore urban district (11% of total population of the state) was chosen as it contained the urban agglomerate of Bangalore, and the Bangalore rural district (3% of the total population of the state) was chosen for its corresponding rural sample. In the case of the other districts, urban and rural districts were chosen within each district. Dakshina Kannada (3% of the total population of the state) on the coast, Davanagere (3% of the total population of the state) in the central region and Bidar (3% of the total population of the state) in the northern arid region were also selected. This yielded eight sampling strata. In order that the final sample be representative of the population distribution in the state, the proportion of men and women in each sampling unit was calculated according to the 2001 Census of India.

Thereafter, in each district, census enumeration blocks were randomly selected. In each block, male and female enumerators sampled every alternate house, with males interviewing male and females interviewing female respondents. In case of refusal or inability to contact after the second visit, enumerators were instructed to move on to the next designated household. On no account were males and females from the same household interviewed. While permission was obtained from the head of household to interview members, subjects were contacted directly and interviewed separately from the family. Enumerators were also instructed to sequentially select the youngest, middle and oldest amongt males and females (in successive families) who satisfied the selection criteria, in case multiple members of any gender in a family did so. In case the quota was not filled up, enumerators moved on to the next randomly selected enumeration block.

A total sample of 3000 male and female respondents was the initial target. However, a few records needed to be discarded because of incomplete or inadequate information, and in at least six cases records were destroyed in heavy rain. The project started in the month of May 2003 and data collection was completed on 30 September 2003.

INSTRUMENTS

The GENACIS core questionnaire developed by IRGGA contains questions about drinking behavior, drinking contexts (where, when, and with whom a person drinks), and drinking consequences (as perceived both by the respondent and by other people), and includes alcohol dependence questions from the Alcohol Use Disorders Identification Test (AUDIT) (Saunders et al., 1993). The questionnaire attempts to assess consumption not only of legal commercial alcoholic beverages but also of illicit or unrecorded alcoholic beverages (e.g., home brew, moonshine, and smuggled alcohol), which in some developing countries constitute most of the alcohol consumed. In addition to measures of alcohol consumption, the GENACIS questionnaire asks about various life domains that may affect or be affected by alcohol use, including social networks and social support, social roles (employment, marriage, parenthood), intimate relationships and sexuality, experiences of violence and victimization, physical and emotional health, use of prescribed and illicit drugs, and excessive or compulsive behavior such as eating or gambling. The study also evaluates the effects of *societal-level* characteristics such as gender inequality, using indicators such as female and male education, employment, income, and political participation (Allamani et al., 2000).

Additionally, a checklist on attitudes to alcohol use, with items relating to acceptance of women drinking, expectancies related to reasons for use, propriety of use in men and women in various circumstances, concepts of drunkenness, and acceptance of behaviors consequent to alcohol-related disinhibition was also administered to half of all the male and female respondents.

ANALYSIS

The first level analysis looked at differences in prevalence, pattern of use and alcohol related consequences between males and females. Another aim of this study was to examine the possibility that recent changes in women's education, employment, social status and economic independence have impacted female drinking patterns. Therefore the second level of analysis examined differences between urban SEC A&B women drinkers and Non-SEC A & B women drinkers [see Box 4].

For this purpose SEC A & B was defined as professionals, semi-

> **Box 4: Socioeconomic classification**
>
> The socioeconomic classification (SEC), used by the market research industry, groups urban Indian households on the basis of education and occupation of the chief wage earner of the household into five segments (SEC A, SEC B, SEC C, SEC D and SEC E households in that order). This classification is more stable than one based on income alone and being reflective of lifestyle is more relevant to the examination of consumption behaviour. 'High' socioeconomic classes refers to SEC A&B, 'mid' socioeconomic class refers to SEC C and 'low' socioeconomic classes refers to SEC D&E.
>
> The chief age earners (CWEs) of the SEC A households work in executive positions, or as industrialists/ businessmen or shop owners. Almost all of them are graduates, post graduates or professionals. CWEs of SEC B households are primarily employed at clerical or supervisory levels or are shopkeepers and industrialists/ businessmen. Less than half are graduates or post graduates, 38% are educated to the 10th or 12th grade, while 13% have had some college education.
>
> (Indian Readership Survey 1998-1999)

professionals, skilled workers and students living in urban areas and/or having educational qualifications of graduation and higher. The Non SEC A&B comprised men and women living in rural areas or urban working class areas who were semi-skilled or unskilled workers, housewives, etc., and who were non-graduates.

RESULTS

A) IN THE TOTAL SAMPLE

SOCIODEMOGRAPHIC DATA

The final sample consisted of 2979 respondents [1508 males; 1471 female], interviewed across the eight urban and rural sampling areas. This works out to a sex ratio of 1000:974, which compared favorably with the census figure of 1000:964. Thirty per cent of the sample was below the poverty line (earned less than Rs. 1700), which is again comparable to the official figure of 33 %. The literacy rate in the sample was 67.7%,

TABLE 1.   General demographic characteristics of the sample by gender (%)

Characteristics	Male [n=1517]	Female [n=1464]
Age - Mean (SD)	32.9 (12.3) years	32.8 (12.4) years
Residence		
Rural	41.8	44.3
Urban	58.2	55.7
Education		
None	22.4	40.5
< 8 years	35.3	28.6
8+ years	42.3	30.8
Religion		
Hindu	75.5	72.8
Muslim	15.2	17.9
Christian	4.9	8.9
Others	4.4	0.4
Marital status		
Married / living with partner	61.7	77.5
Widowed/divorced/separated	2.0	12.5
Never married	36.3	10.0
Income	Rs. 4196.42 (7860.20)	Rs. 4195.46 (8224.40)
Employment		
Working for pay	86.7	35.4
Student	5.6	2.9
Homemaker	1.3	46.2
Parental or pregnancy leave	0.1	
Not working due to illness	1.6	0.2
Retired	1.2	0.1
Voluntarily unemployed for other reasons	1.6	14.4
Involuntarily unemployed	2.0	0.7

comparable to the state census figure of 67.4 %. Similarly the literacy sex ratio was 1000 males to 757 females, comparable to 1000:727 in the population. Women compared unfavorably with men with respect to literacy, employment and in having a greater proportion of widowed, divorced or separated individuals [Table 1].

PREVALENCE OF ALCOHOL USE

Table 2 shows that 5.8 % of all female respondents (86 out of 1471) reported drinking alcohol at least once in the last 12 months, compared to alcohol use in 33.2 % of all male respondents (502 out of 1508). Fifty six per cent of the men and 84% of the women were lifetime abstainers, while 10.5 % of men and 10.1% women reported that they were current abstainers with a history of alcohol use (at least once) in their lifetime.

TABLE 2.   Quantity and frequency of drinking by gender and age[1]

Quantity[2] x Frequency[3]	Males				Females			
	Total (N= 1508)	Grouped by age (%)			Total (N=1471)	Grouped by age (%)		
		Young	Middle aged	Old		Young	Middle aged	Old
Lifetime abstainer	847 (56.2%)	62.6	45.9	57.6	1236 (84.0%)	86.4	83.0	79.7
Ex-drinker	159 (10.5%)	8.8	11.7	13.0	149 (10.1%)	8.4	10.9	13.4
Infrequent light	127 (8.4%)	8.4	9.3	6.9	36 (2.4%)	2.1	2.5	3.3
Frequent light	72 (4.8%)	4.1	5.1	6.2	10 (0.7%)	0.4	0.8	1.1
Infrequent heavy	64 (4.2%)	3.7	6.3	2.2	16 (1.1%)	1.3	0.8	1.1
Frequent heavy	239 (15.8%)	12.5	21.8	14.1	24 (1.6%)	1.5	1.9	1.4

[1] Age categories: Young = 15-29 years; Middle aged = 30-44 years; Old = 45 years and older.
[2] Quantity: Light = less than 5 standard drinks on typical occasions; Heavy = five or more drinks on typical occasions.
[3] Frequency: Lifetime Abstainer = never ever used alcohol; Ex-drinker = no drinking in the past 12 months or more; Infrequent = less frequent than once a weekly; Frequent = drinking once a week or more frequently.

PATTERNS OF DRINKING

QUANTITY AND FREQUENCY

Almost sixteen percent of the male population and two percent of the female population reported frequent (weekly or more) heavy (5+ drinks) drinking. This translates to frequent heavy drinking in 47.6% of male drinkers and 27.9% of female drinkers. Infrequent but heavy drinking was reported by 4.2% of the male population and 1.3% percent of the female population. Effectively then, 46.5% of women drinkers and 60.4% of male drinkers reported heavy drinking on typical drinking occasions [Table 2]. The heavy drinking was prominent in the middle-aged rather than in the younger population among men, but in women this was equally distributed across all age groups.

Female users drank 4.5 (2.4) drinks per typical drinking occasion compared to 5.8 (3.5) drinks consumed by male drinkers. However, the modal value was 6 drinks for both females and males. When the heavy drinkers (people drinking more than six drinks per typical drinking occasion) were removed, there was no significant difference between male and female drinkers (mean of 4 drinks per typical occasion).

Also, after removing the urban center of Bangalore, there was no significant difference between men and women in the quantity of alcoholic beverage drunk per typical drinking occasion [F:M = 5.2 (1.8) drinks : 5.9 (2.7) drinks; t = 7.3, df 74, p= 0.77]. Women drank significantly less often than men [Female: 101 (139.3) days per year, Median = mode = 36 days per year; Male: 154.1 (154.6) days per year, Median = 52 days, mode = 365 days; t = 3, df 581, p = 0.003]. More men (62.1%) than women (39.1%) drank once a week or more often [χ^2 = 16.2, df 1, p < 0.0005].

The total number of drinks (product of number of drinks and number of drinking occasions for each beverage drunk by the individual) was calculated, with the highest frequency in each response category taken as the number of times per year (e.g., 7 to 11 times a year was taken as 11 times per year). Women users drank significantly less [746 (1151) drinks per year; mode 2190 drinks and median 180 drinks; range 2– 4686 drinks per year) than men [1409 (2412) drinks per year; mode 2190 drinks and median 312 drinks; range 1–2295 drinks per year].

Current abstention from alcohol was commoner among rural men than urban men, while it was marginally higher among rural women than among urban women. Current abstainers were roughly equally prevalent among rural and urban women, however rural women had a lower prevalence of lifetime abstainers. A larger proportion of rural than of urban women drinkers reported drinking weekly or more often, as well as drinking 5+ drinks per occasion. In contrast, a larger proportion of urban than of rural male drinkers reported drinking 5+ drinks per occasion, though the proportion of males drinking weekly or more was roughly equal between rural and urban respondents [Table 3].

A common finding in males and females was that both frequent drinking and heavy drinking was more likely in the less educated (eight or less years of formal education), among those who had incomes below the 75th percentile and in those who were married or co-habiting [Table 3].

TABLE 3. Drinking patterns among demographic characteristics (%)

Demographic characteristics	Male				Female			
	All males	Male Drinkers			All females	Female Drinkers		
	Current Abstainers	Frequent drinking[1]	Ever drinks 5+ drinks per day	Heavy drinking[2]	Current Abstainers	Frequent drinking[1]	Ever drinks 5+ drinks per day	Heavy drinking[2]
Residence								
Rural	77.1	63.2	63.9	54.9	95.6	55.2	72.4	58.6
Urban	59.2	61.5	67.9	62.6	93.0	31.6	45.6	40.4
Education								
< 8 years	60.8	73.2	70.5	62.7	95.2	51.4	54.1	45.9
>/= 8 years	70.2	53.2	63.8	58.5	93.1	30.6	55.1	46.9
Marital status								
Married/co-habiting	61.9	64.1	67.8	62.1	95.0	43.9	74.5	54.4
Widowed, separated etc	60.0	50.0	75.0	33.3	91.8	46.7	46.7	40.0
Never married	75.3	57.4	63.2	58.1	90.1	14.3	10.6	21.4
Income								
Lowest 1/4	70.7	65.3	64.3	62.2	96.0	45.0	60.0	55.0
middle 1/2	65.8	62.5	70.3	62.2	94.2	38.5	66.7	51.3
highest 1/4	65.0	57.9	60.3	54.5	91.0	37.0	33.3	33.3
Religion								
Hindu	64.1	65.2	67.4	61.3	94.4	48.3	56.7	51.7
Muslim	86.0	50.0	59.4	59.4	96.5	33.3	88.9	77.8
Christian	57.7	43.3	70.0	46.7	90.8	16.7	41.7	16.7
Multi-denomination	52.5	44.8	58.6	58.6	42.9	0	0	0

[1] Frequent drinking = drinking once a week or more frequently.

[2] Heavy drinking = five or more drinks on typical occasions

Percentages shown for current abstainers are of the total sample in that demographic category (.e.g., rural males). Percentages shown for each pattern of drinking are of the current drinkers in that demographic category. Note that the patterns of drinking are not mutually exclusive.

Heavy drinking and frequent drinking were more common among drinkers from rural areas and drinkers with less education and lower income. This was equally true for male and female drinkers, with the exception of heavy drinking which was more among urban males than rural males. A higher proportion of married drinkers had heavy and frequent drinking compared to unmarried drinkers.

Drinking was also commoner among Hindu, Christian and multi-faith men and women than among Muslims. Christian men and women and men professing faith in multiple religions or agnosticism had a higher prevalence of alcohol use but lower rates of frequent, heavy use.

There was no significant difference between male and female current drinkers in the age at first drink or the duration of drinking.

BEVERAGE OF CHOICE IN DRINKERS

The most common beverage used was spirits (IMFL) in both women (64.3%) and men (70.7%). Nearly fifty per cent of the women users and 53.1% of men users drank beer. Wine was drunk by 27.9% of the drinking women and only 5.6% of the drinking men. Arrack was drunk by 20% of the drinking women and 28.1% of the drinking men. Seven per cent of the drinking women and 7.7% of the drinking men used illicit alcoholic beverages.

Women who drank wine also tended to be more abstemious and drink less (number of drinks per typical drinking occasion) than women who drank spirits, country liquor or illicit liquor [3 (1.7) drinks vs. 5 (2.4) drinks; t = -3.6, df 85, p = 0.001].

Beer-drinking women, on the other hand, drank as much as the women who drank other beverages, unlike beer drinking men who drank less than men drinking other beverages [5.2 (3.6) drinks vs. 6.4 (3.3) drinks; t = -3.6, df 494, p < 0.005]. Arrack drinkers, both men [7.9 (4.3) drinks vs. 5 (2.7) drinks; t = 9, df 494, p < 0.0005] and women [5.8 (2.6) drinks vs. 4.2 (2.3) drinks; t = 0.7, df 22.6, p = 0.03], drank significantly more on typical occasions than those who preferred other beverages.

More than 40% of women restricted themselves to one beverage type, compared to 27% of men. Twenty five per cent of male drinkers drank three or more beverage types across drinking occasions, while 18% of women drinkers did so.

DRINKING CIRCUMSTANCES (see Figure 1)

The most common reported time of drinking (92% of drinking men and 93% of drinking women) was the weekend after 5 p.m.; next most common were weekday evenings after 5 p.m. (81% of men and 76% of women). A larger proportion of drinking men than women drank on weekday evenings [t=2.6, df 106, p=.012]. Of the people who drank daily, an equal proportion of male (20%) and female drinkers (19%) reported drinking everyday or almost everyday in the evening. Thirty two per cent of men and 15% women reported drinking on weekends before 5 p.m. and 25% of men and 13% women reported drinking on weekdays before 5 p.m. (10% and 8% of men and women users reported drinking on weekdays before 5 p.m. daily or almost daily).

Ninety two per cent of drinking men and 93% of drinking women reported that they had never drunk within an hour of driving a vehicle, but this observation needs to be tempered by the fact that a large (unspecified) proportion of the sampled population did not possess or drive vehicles. Women and men spent roughly equal time drinking on a typical day [49.2 (44.8) minutes vs. 41.9 (35.9) minutes; modal value 30 minutes in both groups]. However urban affluent women appeared to spend a longer time on each drink [25 (19) minutes vs. 12.2 (13.8) minutes; t =3.1, df 84, p = 0.003].

Women were more likely to drink with meals [t =5.3, df 105, p<0.0005], at friends' homes [t=5, df104, p<0.0005], at home [t =4.5, df106, p<0.0005], and at parties [t =3.5, df 11.8, p = 0.005]. The men on the other hand were more likely to be drinking at pubs and bars [t =2,

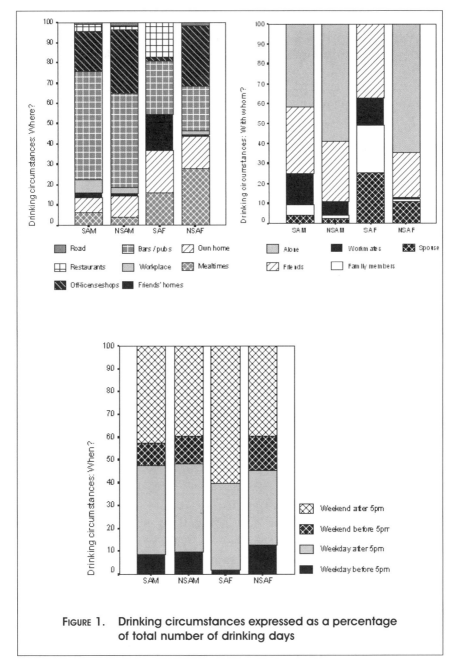

FIGURE 1. **Drinking circumstances expressed as a percentage of total number of drinking days**

df104, p = 0.04], with people from the workplace [t =2.8, df 79, p = 0.006], or drinking alone [t =2.1, df 104, p =.04].

The proportion of individual drinking contexts in relation to the total number of drinking days is illustrated in Figure 1.

HAZARDOUS USE

AUDIT scores were significantly higher among male users than female users [10.4(7.7) vs. 6.8 (5.6); t = 4.1, df 581, p < 0.0005). Male drinkers had consistently higher scores on the individual AUDIT items than female drinkers. Twenty eight per cent of female users and 52% of male users had patterns of use amounting to hazardous drinking [AUDIT $\geq$ 8] (t =4.1, df 551, p < 0.0005).

CONSEQUENCES OF ALCOHOL USE

Among women and men who reported 2 or more problems in the past year (in the areas of work, household chores, physical health, family interaction, finances and legal problems), the women drinkers differed from the men in that they had consumed significantly fewer drinks in the past year [1425.4 (1355) drinks and 3143 (3540) drinks respectively; t = 3.5, df 33.3, p< 0.001].

Similarly, women reporting that their physical health had been poor to fair in the past year drank less frequently than men with the same health status [75(129) days in the past year vs. 218 (158) days in the past year; t = 2.3, df 96, p = 0.02]. They also had a lower mean consumption [776 (1726) drinks per year and 2297 (3103) drinks per year; t = 2.1, df 9.5, p = 0.06], as well as a shorter drinking career [12 (10) years and 17 (13) years; t = 1, df 7.2, p = 0.3], although these differences did not reach statistical significance. More male drinkers (19%) than female drinkers (7%) had faced criticism of their drinking in the past year. Similarly, more male drinkers (10%) than females (1%) admitted that their spouse threatened to leave or left because of their drinking, within the past year.

ALCOHOL AND VIOLENCE

Forty per cent of all males in the total sample and 22% of all women respondents reported solving disagreements by physical fights or long lasting quarrels more than several times a week.

Fifty per cent of the male drinkers and 40% of the female drinkers said that they became more aggressive towards other people after drinking. Twenty seven per cent of female drinkers and only 9% of male drinkers reported that their spouse/partner had been drinking *more often than not, most of the time or all the time* that they had quarreled in the past year. Sixteen per cent of male drinkers and 3% of the female drinkers reported getting into fights after drinking in the past year. Expectedly enough, more male users (45.7%) reported quarreling more than several times a month than male abstainers (35.6%). But among women, there appeared to be an inverse relationship between drinking status and frequent quarreling (2.9% of female users, compared to 5.9% of female abstainers).

Women with alcohol-using spouses (40%) were significantly more likely to have faced violence than women (11%) with abstaining spouses [Pearson Chi-Square = 144.13, df 1, $p < 0.0001$]. Female respondents were also more likely to have been physically aggressive towards alcohol-using spouses (4.5%) than towards abstaining spouses (0.9%) [Pearson Chi-Square=20.38, df1, $p<0.0005$]. However male respondents did not reveal any greater likelihood of physical aggression towards alcohol-using spouses, compared to males with abstaining spouses [Pearson Chi-Square=0.13, df1, $p = 0.72$].

Alcohol-using males were significantly more likely (three times more so) to have been physically aggressive towards their spouses, compared to male abstainers [Pearson Chi-Square = 26.15, df 1, $p < 0.0001$]. Female users were no more likely than female abstainers to have been physically aggressive towards their spouses [Pearson Chi-Square = 0.21, df 1, $p = 0.65$].

EFFECTS OF DRINKING ON INTIMACY AND SEXUALITY

Seventy one per cent of the male users and 58% of female users reported that they found it easier to be open with other people after drinking. Sixty-five per cent of men and 54% of women found it easier to talk to their present partner about their feelings or problems after drinking.

Forty per cent of men and 19% of women felt less inhibited about sex after drinking and 40% of the men and 21% of the women felt that sexual activity was more pleasurable for them after drinking. Likewise about 40% of men and 21% of women felt more sexually attractive after drinking.

Women users reported having their first consensual intercourse at a significantly older age than abstaining women [20(5) years vs. 18.6 (4); $t =$ 2.8, df 1248, $p<0.005$], but there was no significant difference in the number of sexual partners between these two groups. Male users, on the other hand, reported having more sexual partners [0.85 (0.78) vs. 0.65 (.68); $t = 5$, df 1512, $p<0.0005$], but did not differ from abstainers in age at first sexual intercourse. The male heavy users accounted for this effect, as they had significantly more sexual partners than light users and abstainers [0.92(0.85) vs. 0.66(0.67); $t = 5.9$, df 203, $p < 0.0005$].

ALCOHOL AND OTHER SUBSTANCES

More alcohol-using women used tobacco (36%) than non-using women. Similarly, male alcohol users were more likely to use tobacco (51%) than non users (34%). The prevalence of prescription drug abuse was three times higher in women users (2.4%) than non-users (0.7%). On the other hand, use of these substances was relatively higher among male non-users (9.5%) than users (7.9%).Although the general prevalence was very low, use of cannabis was higher among both alcohol-using women and men (1.2% and 1.4%) than in the general population of women and men (0.1% and 0.2%). The prevalence of gambling was similarly three times higher among women users (1.2 %) than non-users (0.3%). Gambling was also higher among male users (5.8 %) than non-users (1.9%).

Age at onset of alcohol use : There was no significant difference in age at onset of use between male and female users [20.7 (5.3) years and 20.3 (5.9) years respectively]. Younger alcohol users, both male [Pearson Correlation = 0.37, p < 0.0005] and female [Pearson Correlation = 0.34, p < 0.0005] were significantly more likely to have an earlier age at onset of use. Males over 35 years had a mean age at onset of use of 22.5 (6.2) years, compared to 19.5 (4.2) years in users currently below 35 years [t = 6.4, df 492, p < 0.005]. Women users over 35 years had a mean age at onset of use of 22 (6.7) years, compared to 19.1 (5.4) years in users currently below 35 years [t = 2.2, df 79, p < 0.03].

COURSE : LIFE CYCLE AND USE

Among women, there was a significantly negative correlation between age and quantity drunk per typical occasion (Pearson Correlation = - 0.27, p = 0.016) and with frequency of six or more drinks drunk per typical occasion (Pearson Correlation = - 0.26, p = 0.026). This was not observed in male drinkers.

INFLUENCES ON DRINKING

Thirty-five per cent of female users had alcohol-using spouses, compared to 3% of male drinkers. Ten per cent of female users reported that all or most drinking occasions in the past year had been with their spouse or partner, compared to only 1.6% of male users, yet only 4% of married female users reported having felt influenced to drink by their spouse.

Twelve per cent of all women respondents and 7.7% of all male respondents reported childhood sexual abuse by close family members and 3.9% and 3.5% respectively, by others. The occurrence of childhood sexual abuse [CSA] was disproportionately higher among women users [20.5% vs. 11.3%; x^2=5.7, p = 0.017) than female abstainers. But the history of CSA did not appear to influence heavy use or bingeing in men or women.

Forcible sex after the age of 16 years was present in 10.4% of all women respondents and 1.6% of all males. Ninety-five percent of women and 54% of the men so abused had suffered at the hands of a close relative, spouse or partner. However, none of the women users reported such incidents in the past year.

ATTITUDES TOWARDS DRINKING

An equal proportion of abstaining and alcohol-using women (54%) agreed strongly that it was more acceptable for men to drink than women. However that left more than 45% of women in both groups who disagreed strongly with that contention. A disproportionate number (75.8%) of the women who disagreed were from an urban background [χ^2=24, df 1, p < 0.0005]. Among women who agreed with this contention there was no difference between rural and urban residents. A significantly larger number of men than women (irrespective of drinking status) [63% vs 54%; χ^2=9.7, df 1, p = 0.002] disapproved of women drinking.

Women users were significantly more likely than women abstainers to agree that it is acceptable for women to drink in private or when accompanied by the husband or other male relatives [48% vs. 31%; χ^2=3.9, df1, p = 0.049]. Ninety per cent of all males strongly rejected that notion, compared to 52% of all females [χ^2=25.5, df1, p < 0.0005]. Eighty-five percent of abstaining women and 38% of drinking women expected that women were much more likely than men to experience physical problems with alcohol [χ^2=31.6, df1, p < 0.0005]. This expectancy was more common in all women (83%), irrespective of drinking status, than in the men (75%) [χ^2= 9, df1, p = 0.003].

Abstaining women were significantly more likely than using women to anticipate that women were much more likely than men to experience emotional problems with alcohol [χ^2= 35, df1, p < 0.0005]. Men (78%) were in fact less open to this possibility than women (83%), though the difference was statistically non-significant. More women than men agreed that men were more likely to get violent after drinking [χ^2=5.9, df1, p = 0.02]. Significantly more men (68%) than women (42%) expressed the opinion that it was really no point having a drink if one did not feel high at the end of it [χ^2=50, df1, p < 0.0005].

ATTRIBUTIONS: REASONS FOR DRINKING

The items on the Attitudes questionnaire pertaining to expectancies governing reasons for drinking were grouped into two subscales: 1] Drinking to enhance positive experiences and 2] drinking to relieve stress and tension. Male drinkers had significantly higher scores [t = 3.3, df 256, p = 0.001] on the former than women, but did not differ on the tension relief subscale.

B) SEC A & B MEN AND WOMEN

Since the available background information as well as the first level of analyses appeared to suggest that this group had a significantly different spectrum of alcohol use, a separate analysis was done for men and women representing this group.

SOCIODEMOGRAPHIC DATA

SEC A & B men and women comprised 21% of the urban sample. This is similar to the estimate of 28% in the SEC A & B segment in urban India

(Indian Readership Survey 1998-1999). Women comprised 25% of the SEC A & B group (90 of 355) and 52% of the Non- SEC A & B group (1374 of 2626).

PREVALENCE OF ALCOHOL USE

Nearly nineteen per cent of SEC A & B women [SAF] (17 of 90) were current drinkers, compared to 5% of the Non- SEC A & B women [NSAF](70 of 1374). The prevalence of current drinking was 41.5% and 30.8% among SEC A & B men [SAM] and non- SEC A & B men [NSAM] respectively. SAF women had a four times greater prevalence of alcohol use than NSAF women. SAF drinkers were significantly younger [t =2.9, df 60.8, p = 0.004], more educated [t = 7, df 23.2, p < 0.0005] and earned more than NSAF drinkers. They were also better educated than SAM consumers [t = 4.6, df 13, p<0.0005].

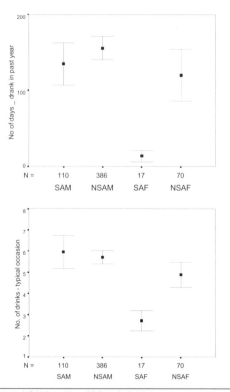

SAM = SEC A & B Males; NSAM = Non SEC A & B Males;
SAF = SEC A & B Females; NSAF = Non SEC A & B Females.
See Box 3 for details of these categories.

SEC A & B Females significantly drank less frequently and had less drinks per typical drinking occasion. The quantity and frequency of Non SEC A & B Females were nearer to that observed in male drinkers.

FIGURE 2.   **Quantity and Frequency of Drinking - SEC A&B vs. Non-SEC A&B**

PATTERNS OF USE : QUANTITY AND FREQUENCY

There was no significant difference between SEC A& B [SAM] and Non-SEC A & B men [NSAM] with respect to frequency of drinking, number of drinks on typical occasions, or total consumption in a year. SEC A & B women [SAF] drank significantly less, in terms of number of drinks in past year [t = -2.7, df 85, p = 0.008] and had a shorter mean duration of alcohol use [statistically non-significant] than non-SEC A & B women [NSAF] (Figure 2). There was no significant difference between SEC A & B and Non-SEC A & B men with respect to frequency of drinking, number of drinks on typical occasions, or total consumption in a year.

PATTERNS OF USE: BEVERAGE OF CHOICE

Spirit drinkers: Women who drank spirits, drank significantly less spirits than male spirit drinkers [4.4 (2.2) drinks vs. 6.1 (3.8) drinks per typical occasion; t = 4.9, df 415, p < 0.0005]. The difference appears to have been contributed by SEC A&B women, as there was no significant difference between non-SEC A&B women and all male drinkers [Figure 2].

Wine drinkers: The increased prevalence of use of wine by women consumers was predominantly due to SEC A&B women. SEC A&B women consumers had had more wine drinking days [t = 3.6, df 82, p = 0.001], and had fewer days when they drank spirits (a mean of 16 days in the year, compared to 110 days in men) [t = 6, df101, p<0.0005] or even beer (mean of 12 days in the year vs. 28 days in men; t = 2, df30, p<0.048).

DIFFERENCES IN DRINKING CIRCUMSTANCES

SEC A & B women were more likely than the other women to drink at restaurants [t = 7.2, df 84, p < 0.0005], parties [t = 6.5, df 84, p<0.0005], friends' homes [t = 3.8, df 83, p<0.0005], in their own homes [t =2.3, df 78, p = 0.02] and drink along with meals (statistically non-significant). They also differed from the non-SEC A & B women, in that they were more likely to drink with friends [t = 5.7, df 24.7, p<0.0005], and to drink along with family members other than their spouse [t =3.6, df 83, p = 0.001] and with people from their workplace [t = 2.9, df 82, p<0.005]. They were significantly less likely to drink alone [t = -4.4, df 65, p < 0.0005]. Solitary drinking was significantly more observed among rural women ($\chi2$= 4.3, df 1, p = 0.03) and men ($\chi2$= 5.4, df 1, p = 0.02) compared to their urban counterparts. SEC A & B women appeared to spend a longer time on each drink [25 (19) minutes vs. 12.2 (13.8) minutes; t = 3.1, df 84, p = 0.003]. [See Figure 2]

PATTERNS OF USE: HAZARDOUS USE

A significantly lesser number of female users (28%) compared to male users (52%) had patterns of use amounting to hazardous drinking [AUDIT

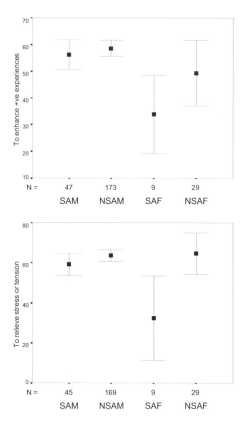

FIGURE 3. Reasons for drinking

$\geq$ 8] (t=4.1, df 551, p < 0.0005). SEC A&B females were significantly less likely to have hazardous drinking compared to non-SEC A&B females (t =- 2.9, df 85, p=0.005).

LIFE CYCLE AND USE

The quantity of alcohol drunk significantly decreased with advancing age, (Pearson Correlation = - 0.35, p = 0.003), along with the duration of drinking (Pearson Correlation = - 0.35, p = 0.003), among the non-SEC A&B women. There was no such relationship observed among the SEC A & B women. In this group, on the other hand. the duration of drinking correlated significantly (Pearson Correlation = 0.64, p = 0.006) with the number of drinking days in the past year as well as with number of drinks in the past year (Pearson Correlation = 0.91, p < 0.0005). SEC A & B women drinking for 7 years or more were more likely to be drinking multiple beverages than those who had shorter drinking careers.

ATTRIBUTIONS: REASONS FOR DRINKING

Among women drinkers, the non-SEC A&B women had significantly higher scores than the SEC A&B women on drinking for tension relief, but not for enhancement of positive expectancies.

DISCUSSION

PREVALENCE

It comes as no surprise that alcohol use in women in the state of Karnataka in southern India is much lower than the prevalence in men. This is not dissimilar to previous observations from India (Benegal et al., 2003; Saxena, 1999; Isaac, 1998), which have reported a significantly lower prevalence of alcohol use among women compared to men. This is also similar to observations throughout the world, across different cultural contexts of drinking.

Why do women drink less than the men? The obvious answer is that it is socio-culturally less acceptable; the prevailing sentiment, and one that appears to be traditionally held since ancient times, is that it is more acceptable for men to drink than for women. This is inextricably linked to the woman's position in society and is buttressed by strong associations with morality. There is expectedly a strong male gender bias against women drinking (even among men who themselves use alcohol). Rural women and the urban poor [the Non-SEC A&B], continued to support the status quo, even the drinkers among them. Women from urban areas with professional, semiprofessional or skilled jobs and students were more permissive and tolerant of women's drinking, regardless of drinking status. This group predictably had a higher prevalence of drinking.

Also, women, much more than men, believed that alcohol was more likely to cause physical and emotional problems in women than men. A larger proportion of abstaining than of drinking women endorsed this belief. Such a health belief model (Kauffman, Silver & Poulin, 1997) is likely to shape drinking choices in women. It has been observed earlier that such negative expectancies about health consequences are likely to prevent or temper use (Green et al., 2003). The 6% prevalence of drinking in adult women (vs. 33% of men) is relatively higher than that recorded in a previous study from this region, which indicated a prevalence of less than 2% (Benegal et al., 2003). At one level this is related to the sampling design in this study, which gave greater weight to the population in the urban center of Bangalore, which has the maximum population density in the region. The previous study had used a stratified sampling design with an equal proportion of respondents from all the five districts involved, without regard to the actual population density. This underestimated the drinkers in the urban SEC A&B group. In the current assessment, the urban working class women and the rural women drinkers [Non-SEC A&B]

constituted 2% of all adult women, with the urban affluent women drinkers group adding a further 4%. The relatively higher prevalence is also due to the fact that the sampling scheme in this study involved approaching male and female respondents directly. Previous studies usually involved approaching respondents nominated by the head of the household as drinkers or non-drinkers. Given the prevailing social attitudes to alcohol use, this obviously led to lower estimates of female users.

The prevalence of alcohol use, then, is almost twice as high among urban women from middle and upper socioeconomic backgrounds. Again, this is a departure from earlier findings; studies done ten to twenty years back generally reported that rural and tribal women, or women from a lower socioeconomic urban milieu, had a relatively higher prevalence of use. SEC A&B women had shorter drinking careers than women from rural and lower socioeconomic backgrounds, indicating that there were a large number of recent users in this group. 50% of the former had drinking careers of less than 10 years, compared to only 20% of the latter. This could possibly be a snapshot of an ongoing change in drinking habits among urban women of middle and upper socioeconomic status.

PATTERNS OF DRINKING

Taking the trends for the entire state, women drank significantly less than men on typical drinking occasions (although the modal value of drinks per typical occasion was six drinks in both men and women). However, if the women in the urban center of Bangalore are omitted from the analysis, there is no difference between men and women with respect to amounts drunk on a typical drinking occasion. This is similar to observations recorded earlier in this region, which highlighted the fact that women drank as much as men when they did drink (Benegal et al., 2003). In fact, at a mean of five standard drinks consumed on typical drinking occasions, both women and men qualified for a pattern of bingeing whenever they drank at all. This can be considered the traditional pattern of drinking among Indian women.

The consumption was significantly lower and different among women from upper and middle socioeconomic groups, especially in the larger urban centres and the increasingly *globalized* city of Bangalore. Women, however, drank less frequently than men. In the men, daily drinking was the predominant pattern (around 60%); but while daily drinking in women users was significantly less, it was still the pattern reported by 40% of the women users.

This translates into a lower annual consumption in women. Nevertheless, keeping in mind the trend for bingeing on every occasion, this still is a very explosive pattern of drinking, albeit relatively less frequent than the men's. It is well appreciated (Heath, 2000; Stockwell et al, 1996) that binge drinking and drinking to intoxication are associated with more adverse consequences, particularly acute consequences. Both women and men appeared to be consuming large quantities of alcohol in a very short time. Drinking five to six drinks in about half an hour can lead to very high Blood Alcohol levels, which in turn is likely to predispose to greater morbidity. The SEC A&B woman, however, appeared to prefer sipping her drink rather than gulping it down, in a departure from the overall trend.

It is not surprising, then, that almost a third of women users and a half of male users had patterns of alcohol use amounting to hazardous drinking. In keeping with the general trend, the SEC A&B women were less likely to display patterns of hazardous drinking. Previous studies, from all over India, have similarly observed that one out of two people who drink alcohol do so at hazardous levels. Benegal (2003) documented that around 50% of women users and around 70% of male users had hazardous use. Compared to other Asian cultures, like Thailand (27% in males and 1% in females; Assangkornchai et al., 2003), this is abnormally high.

As such, it seems evident that there is a bi-modal distribution of female alcohol use. One pattern is seen predominantly in urban, relatively affluent, more educated women who are students or higher paid working women (professionals, semi-professionals and skilled workers). A second pattern is seen amongst rural or urban working class women, who were mainly housewives or working in low income unskilled jobs. It appears likely, that here, different patterns of alcohol use are supplanting traditional patterns. In the hinterland, the traditional patterns continue.

Women users suffered equivalent physical health consequences to males at lower quantities and frequencies. There is also a suggestion from this data that physical consequences occurred after a shorter duration of drinking than in the men, and that women are prone to more rapid progression of alcohol-related health problems. This is entirely consistent with the *telescoping* of alcohol-related physical consequences which has often been observed in women alcoholics (Redgrave, 2003; Greenfield, 2002). Alcohol use, as in males, constituted for females yet another node in a matrix of risk. Women alcohol users were also likely to have other high-risk lifestyle issues. Tobacco use (smoking and smokeless) was significantly more common among alcohol users than abstainers, with more than a third of all drinking women using tobacco. Expectedly, tobacco use was higher in males compared to women.

Prescription drug abuse was also three times higher among women users than women abstainers. In contrast, the prevalence of such abuse was higher in abstinent males compared to users. It has been observed also in other cultures that women tend to use more medically prescribed psychotropics than men (Grant et al., 2004; Canetto, 1999); however, in the present sample males as a whole used more psychotropics. One wonders if male abstainers are "substituting" prescription drugs for alcohol in an environment where alcohol use is generally stigmatized.

Use of other substances was low, with cannabis use at about 1% in both males and females using alcohol. The prevalence among non-drinkers was rare. It has been repeatedly observed that in southern India, in contradistinction to the north and north-eastern parts of the country, substance use other than alcohol is very low (Rapid Assessment Survey of Drug Abuse in India, 2002).

Gambling was higher among female users than female abstainers, but on the whole far lower than among male users.

COHORT EFFECTS

Although there appeared to be no difference between men and women with respect to the age at which they started drinking, there was a significant lowering of age at onset of alcohol use among men and women in later birth cohorts. This is again consistent with data from a previous study from the same region that found very strong cohort effects, with an accelerated onset of regular use of alcohol in younger birth cohorts (Benegal et al., 2003).

EFFECTS OF AGE

A major gender related difference was the trend towards lower alcohol use (number of drinks on typical drinking occasions) with increasing age in non SEC A&B women. Men, conversely, tended to drink more with increasing age. SEC A&B women appeared to be at greater risk of increasing consumption with increasing duration of drinking. This raises the likelihood that they too will in time have similarly explosive patterns of drinking as their non-SEC A&B counterparts, even though their current consumption is low. While the newly introduced low alcohol ready-to-drink beverages do not figure in this analysis, there is the very real possibility that the SEC A&B women who start off with ready-to-drink beverages (pre-mixed drinks) or wine will shift to stronger alcoholic beverages. There is some evidence that this process is already happening. SEC A & B women who have been drinking for 7 years or more are drinking multiple beverages, as well as drinking more frequently and larger quantities than those with shorter drinking careers.

PREFERRED BEVERAGES

It has been consistently recorded by previous observers that spirits are the preferred alcoholic beverage in India (Benegal, 2003; Saxena, 1999; Isaac, 1998) and this is borne out in the present study. Spirits [Indian Made Foreign Liquors] were the most common beverage among both men and women in both urban and rural areas. Beer was next common beverage in both men and women, regardless of urban or rural milieu. This is a departure from previous studies which have consistently shown a low consumption of beer in India. However, this parallels the growing trends in beer sales (especially strong beer) over the past few years. Arrack (country liquor) was the next most commonly used beverage, but concentrated entirely in the Non-SEC A&B segment. Arrack appears to be less common among women, though. Illicit (moonshine) liquor was common in rural areas and among urban working class women. In fact it was more popular among women than men. We have previously documented that in urban working class areas and in rural areas, where illicit liquor outlets abound and are merged with the surroundings, it is easier for women in these circumstances to acquire their drink without attracting unwelcome attention (Benegal, 2003).

Whether they drank illicit liquor, arrack, or beer, women and men drank similar amounts. A notable exception were women from the SEC A&B segment who, when drinking spirits, drank significantly smaller amounts than the men. A significantly higher proportion of women admitted drinking wine than the men, and this was mostly among the SEC A&B segment. Wine- drinking women tended to be more abstemious.

More women than men restricted themselves to one beverage type. Men on the other hand were more catholic in their beverage choice and tended to drink multiple beverages.

DRINKING CIRCUMSTANCES

Weekend drinking (after 5 p.m.) was the most frequent event for both men and women. An equal proportion of men and women users reported drinking every evening or almost every evening. This accounted for a fifth of both male and female users. But regular heavy drinking, probably qualifying for alcohol dependence, was also common. Almost a tenth of male and female users, respectively, drank on weekdays before 5 p.m. daily or almost daily. Women and men spent roughly equal time (around half an hour) drinking on typical occasions.

More than a third of all female users had alcohol-using spouses and a tenth of the women users drank almost exclusively along with their spouses. This observation is a validation of earlier findings, where it was noted that most alcohol-using women were strongly influenced by significant males in the family (spouses, fathers, brothers) in initiation and patterns of drinking.

The impact of male alcohol use on women and children has been a major focus of attention in the public discourse on alcohol in India. In fact this aspect found repeated mention in the debates of the Constituent Assembly in 1950 when the founding fathers of the modern Indian republic debated and endorsed prohibition as a Directive Principle of state policy, repeatedly underlining the effects of alcohol on violence towards women and children and on poverty. It has also been at the root of several women's anti-alcohol movements, which have culminated in well publicized but short-lived attempts at prohibition in a few states in the country. Women with alcohol-using spouses, in this study, were much more likely to have faced acts of physical violence than women with abstaining spouses. The converse did not hold true, as women alcohol users were no more likely than abstaining women to be violent towards their spouses.

In the general population, there was a strong expectancy linking alcohol use and the propensity to violence in men, rather than in women. This was more common among women. Intoxication as a desired outcome of drinking was a stronger expectancy among men than in women. This was in line with the other male belief, that men tend to get drunk more than women. In combination, this set of expectancies is likely to be a powerful template that legitimizes male drunkenness and violence after drinking.

A glance at the city page of any newspaper in India will underscore this point. On any day there are invariably one or more gory reports of murder and mayhem perpetrated by drunken men. Sometimes there are reports of long-suffering wives or parents striking back. There is evidence of this, too, from the present study's findings. Alcohol-using males were at greater risk of violence from their spouses, compared to abstaining men. Surprisingly, despite the proscriptive attitudes towards alcohol use in women, women users appeared to be at no greater risk for suffering spousal violence than abstaining women. If at all, they appeared to be at lesser risk. This finding must be treated with caution.

WOMEN DRINKERS

To sum up, there appear to be two widely divergent patterns of drinking among women. There is what appears to be a traditional pattern, as reported earlier. This is confined to less educated women from rural settings and poorer sections of urban society. Their drinking is marked by bingeing and drinking to intoxication, with a high proportion drinking five drinks or more per drinking occasion. This pattern is marked by predominant use of cheaper, high alcohol-containing beverages: spirits, illicit liquor and country liquor. Drinking is mostly conducted in under-socialized drinking contexts. This group is more likely to drink at home, usually alone. They are also more likely to drink at off-license retail outlets, and licensed retail outlets like arrack shops. Though they drink less frequently, their pattern is nearer the male pattern of drinking observed in the sample. It also appears to be more likely to serve the function of tension relief rather than the enhancement of positive experiences. Drinking to enhance positive experiences appears to be less of a motivation for women as a whole compared to males. It is reasonable to posit that relief of negative emotional states rather than the pursuit of pleasure appears to be the dominant motif driving women's drinking, especially among women from lower socioeconomic groups. It is clearly ego-dystonic, and leaves a lot of guilt and shame in its wake. They also report more alcohol-related problems in the sphere of household chores, relations with family and children, physical health, family finances and friendships.

Then there is the other pattern, seen in affluent, educated urban women who are presumably more emancipated. This group is comparatively younger, more educated, earn more, drink less on typical drinking occasions, less frequently and have a shorter duration of drinking. They are more likely to be unmarried and without children. Their drinking is under relatively more socialized circumstances: at restaurants, parties, with spouses, family members, workmates and friends. It is more normalized in that they are more likely to drink at home and with meals. Although spirit drinking is still most common, use of lower alcoholic beverages like wine and beer is relatively higher. Women's drinking is perceived to be more socially acceptable in this group (although it does not really have significantly more male endorsement). Women in this group are motivated equally by expectancies of tension relief and the enhancement of positive experiences. These women obviously have a much higher spending capacity. They also have less physical, emotional and interpersonal problems as a result of their drinking. This group is characterized by people in their early drinking careers, and there are suggestions that the newer entrants are starting to drink at progressively younger ages. This is so different from the traditional pattern of women's drinking that some observers have suggested that a novel, convivial (westernized) pattern is supplanting older drinking norms.

In marketing terms they represent two different markets. The rural and poorer urban consumers, who drink mostly non-premium spirits and country liquor, constitute a market which is comparatively stagnant. The young, affluent female urban drinker conversely represents an emerging market, which is rapidly growing. And this is clearly recognized by local alcohol manufacturers and trans-national alcoholic beverage corporations. According to one influential industry projection which predicts a realistic market growth of 12-14% of beverage alcohol sales in India for the next ten years, increasing drinking among women is expected to fuel over a quarter of that movement.

The president of one of India's largest beverage alcohol manufacturing companies, in a television interview, confirmed that *"the entire Indian market is changing...[with] a huge explosion of disposable income among the young. Moreover, social drinking has increased. The Indian market is ready for ready to drink [RTD] alcohol beverages with exotic fruit flavors...which will be a stepping stone for SEC A [urban higher income] youngsters and women to enter the alcoholic beverages segment. Especially women, who are used to fruit juices and would readily make the transition to one with low alcohol content* ("Speak" programme on SAB TV). Ready- to-drink or mixed beverages (RTD), introduced into the Indian market in 2001, have in a short span of time found a substantial market amongt urban youth and women. The wine market, again targeted at women, is growing at 25% per year (from 0.6 million bottles sold in 1997 to 2 million bottles in 2002).

LIMITATIONS OF THE STUDY

It must be admitted that some of the observations made in this paper are based on very small sample sizes. The generalizations on women's drinking are after all based on just 87 women. The women in the SEC A&B segment number only seventeen.

But it is undeniable that the prevalence of women's drinking in India is very low. The sample we have gathered is fairly representative of the general population in the state with regard to sex ratio, literacy rates, income, and the proportion of the SEC A&B segment. Moreover, these figures seem to duplicate earlier findings from the same population, with the exception of the prevalence of drinking in women. And there appears to be a logical explanation for that discrepancy. Also, the data is regional and can never be taken as being representative of the entire country. However, one must also acknowledge that this is the first such epidemiological data on women's drinking from India. The findings underscore the necessity for planning further studies in this area throughout the country as they have grave public health implications.

It is interesting to contrast two different socio-political trends that appear to have influenced the way alcohol is viewed and used in India. First, there is the phenomenon termed *sanskritisation*, where as a result of social and economic mobility, people of lower socioeconomic class adopt the mores of the higher castes and classes (Srinivas1997). It has been speculated that, with increasing education and urbanization and the resultant social and economic mobility which saw the growth of the urban middle classes in India in the last 150 years or less, there have been rapid changes in diet (in favour of the upper caste Brahminical norms of vegetarianism and abstinence from alcohol) as lower castes/classes adopted the cultural mores of the higher castes/classes in order to better adapt to their changed positions in the social hierarchy. Historically, this has served to push temperance as the stated position on alcohol in the upper and growing middle classes. Alcohol use, in this view, was seen as an atavistic trait of the primitive (tribals and the socially backward) or an aberration/affectation of the upper classes. Among males, even in recent times, although the use of alcohol use has dramatically increased, consumption has been more prevalent among the lower socioeconomic groups than among the middle and upper socioeconomic group [Benegal, 2003].

The results that we observe among women appear to run counter to this trend. Emancipation as a result of education, economic independence and urbanization, along with the effects of globalization that affect women in urban India, appear to increase the chance of initiating alcohol consumption and rapidly increasing the consumer base. As noted earlier, the alcohol industry is well seized of this notion. In most developed economies, at least in Europe, the phenomenon of convergence is as much due to a reduction in male drinking as an increase in female consumption. The real danger in India is that burgeoning consumption in both males and females, encouraged by increasingly permissive social attitudes to alcohol use, pushed by targeted hard-sell by the liquor industry and shaped by the explosive drinking norms, is likely to increase manifold the alarmingly high social cost of alcohol abuse (Benegal et al., 2000) in the country.

ACKNOWLEDGEMENTS

We acknowledge the contributions of Lakshmi Shankaran (Field co-ordinator of the India site) and the field investigators in the GENACIS-India project, Dr. Mala Ramachandran (Bangalore City Corporation), Mrs. Geetha Krishnan; Mr. H. Shashidhar (Director, Census Operations, Karnataka).

REFERENCES

Allamani, A., Voller, F., Kubicka, L., & Bloomfield, K.(2000). Drinking cultures and the position of women in nine European countries. *Subst Abuse, 21*(4), 231-247.

Assanangkornchai, S., Pinkaew, P., & Apakupakul, P. (2003). Prevalence of hazardous-harmful drinking in a southern Thai community. *Drug & Alcohol Review, 22*, 287-293.

Benegal, V., Gururaj, G., & Murthy, P. (2003). Report on a WHO collaborative project on unrecorded consumption of alcohol in Karnataka, India [monograph on the Internet]. Available at http://www.nimhans.kar.nic.in/Deaddiction/lit/UNDOC_Review.pdf

Benegal, V., Gururaj, G., & Murthy, P. (2002). Project report on a WHO multi centre collaborative project on Establishing and Monitoring Alcohol's Involvement in Casualties: 2000-2001 [monograph on the Internet]. Available at http://www.nimhans.kar.nic.in/Deaddiction/lit/Alcohol%20and%20%20Injur ies_WHO%20Collab.pdf

Benegal, V., Shantala, A., Murthy, P., & Janakiramaiah, N. (2001). Report on Development of a Model District Programme for Prevention of Drug and Alcohol Problems: WHO–NIMHANS Project. [monograph on the Internet]. Available at http://www.nimhans.kar.nic.in/Deaddiction/lit/Mandya_distt_WHO.pdf

Benegal, V., Velayudhan, A., & Jain, S. (2000). Social Costs of Alcoholism: A Karnataka Perspective. *NIMHANS Journal, 18* (1&2), 6-7

Bhatt, R. V. (1998). Domestic violence and substance abuse. *International Journal of Gynaecology and Obstetrics 63* Suppl 1, 25-31.

Blume, S. B. (1997). Women and alcohol: Issues in social policy. In Wilsnack, R.W., & Wilsnack, S.C., (eds.), *Gender and alcohol: individual and social perspectives.* New Brunswick, NJ: Rutgers Center of Alcohol Studies (pp. 462–489).

Census of India (2001). Karnataka: provisional population totals – rural urban distribution of population, Paper 2 of 2001. Director of Census Operations, Bangalore, 2001.

Chandra, P. S., Krishna, V. A., Benegal, V., & Ramakrishna, J. (2003). High-risk sexual behaviour and sensation seeking among heavy alcohol users. *Indian Journal of Medical Research,* **117**, 88-92.

Chitra, S., Ashok, L., Anand, L., Srinivasan, V., & Jayanthi, V. (2004). Risk factors for esophageal cancer in Coimbatore, Southern India: a hospital-based case-control study. *Indian Journal of Gastroenterology,* **23**, 117-118

DH News Service Bangalore (2003) Women addicted to alcohol seek help later than men. *Deccan Herald*, Bangalore edition, Thursday, July 31, 2003.

Fillmore, K., Golding, J., Leino, E., Motoyoshi, M., Shoemaker, C., Terry, H., Ager, C., & Ferrer, H. (1997). Patterns and trends in women's and men's drinking. In Wilsnack, R., & Wilsnack, S. (eds.). *Gender and alcohol: individual and social perspectives.* New Brunswick, NJ: Rutgers Center of Alcohol Studies (pp. 21-48).

Doniger, W. (1992). *The Laws of Manu.* New Delhi: Penguin Classics.

Gaunekar, G., Patel, V., Jacob, K. S., Vankar, G., Mohan, D., Rane, A., Prasad, S., Johari, N., & Chopra, A. (2004). Drinking patterns of hazardous drinkers: a multicentre study in India. In Haworth, A., & Simpson, R. (eds.), *Moonshine markets: issues in unrecorded alcohol beverage production and consumption.* New York: Brunner-Routledge (pp.125-144).

Gomberg, E. (1996). Women's drinking practices and problems from a lifespan perspective. In Howard, J., Martin, S., Mail, P., Hilton, M., & Taylor, E. (eds.), *Women and alcohol: issues for prevention research.* National Institute on Alcohol Abuse and Alcoholism (NIAAA) Research Monograph No. 32. NIH Publication No. 96-3817. Bethesda, MD: NIAAA (pp. 185-214).

Grant, M., & Litvak, J. (eds., 1998). *Drinking patterns and their consequences.* Philadephia: Brunner and Mazel.

Green, C. A., Polen, M. R., & Perrin, N. A. (2003). Structural models of gender, alcohol consumption and health. *Substance Use and Misuse,* **38**, 97-125.

Greenfield, S. F. (2002). Women and alcohol use disorders. *Harvard Rev Psychiatry,* **10**, 76-85

Gupta, P. C., Saxena, S., Pednekar, M. S., Maulik, P. K. (2003). Alcohol consumption among middle-aged and elderly men: a community study from western India. *Alcohol and Alcoholism,* **38**, 327-331.

Gururaj, G.(2002). Epidemiology of traumatic brain injuries: Indian scenario. *Neurology Research,* **24**, 24-8.

Gururaj, G., Isaac, M. (2001). Epidemiology of suicides in Bangalore City. NIMHANS Publication No. 43, Bangalore, p.34.

Heath, D. B. (2000). *Drinking occasions: comparative perspectives on alcohol and culture.* Philadelphia, Pennsylvania: Brunner/Mazel.

Hibell, B., Andersson, B., Ahlström, S., Balakireva, O., Bjarnason, T., Kokkevi, A., Morgan M. & Narusk, A. (2001). *The 1999 ESPAD Report: Alcohol and other Drug Use among students in 30 Countries,* Stockholm: Swedish Council for Information on Alcohol and other Drugs.

Holman, C. D., English, D. R., Bower, C., Kurinczuk, J. J. (1996). NHMRC recommendations on abstinence from alcohol in pregnancy. National Health and Medical Research Council. *Medical Journal of Australia,* **164**(11), 699.

Hommer, D., Momenan, R., Kaiser, E., & Rawlings, R. (2001) Evidence for a gender-related effect of alcoholism on brain volumes. *Am J Psychiatry,* **158**(2), 198-204.

Ilaiah, K. (1992). Andhra Pradesh's anti-liquor movement. *Economic and Political Weekly,* **26**(45), 2406-2408.

Isaac, M. (1998). Contemporary trends: India. In Grant, M. (ed.), *Alcohol and emerging markets: patterns, problems and responses*. Baltimore: Taylor and Francis (pp. 145-176).

Jain, A., Buddhiraja, S., Khurana, B., Singhal, R., Nair, D., Arora, P., Gangwal, P., Mishra, S. K., Uppal, B., Gondal, R., & Kar, P. (1999). Risk factors for duodenal ulcer in north India. *Tropical Gastroenterology* **20**, 36-9.

Kauffman, S. E., Silver, P., & Poulin, J. (1997). Gender differences towards alcohol, tobacco and other drugs. *Social Work*, **42**, 231-241.

Kaufman, K. G., & Asdigian, N. (1997).Gender differences in alcohol-related spousal aggression. Wilsnack R and Wilsnack S (Eds.). *Gender and alcohol: individual and social perspectives*. New Brunswick, NJ: Rutgers Center of Alcohol Studies (pp. 312-334).

Kraus, L., Bloomfield, K., Augustin, R., & Reese, A. (2000). Prevalence of alcohol use and the association between onset of use and alcohol related problems in a general population sample in Germany. *Addiction*, **95**(9),1389-1401.

Kumar, V. S. (1997). Behavioural malignancy: alcoholism, a bleak future? In Azariah, J., Azariah, H., & Macer, D. R.J. (eds.), *Bioethics in India: proceedings of the international bioethics workshop in Madras*: Biomanagement of Biogeoresources, 16-19 Jan. 1997, University of Madras. Eubios Ethics Institute. http://www.biol.tsukuba.ac.jp/~macer/index.html

Mahal, A. (2000). What works in alcohol policy? Evidence from rural India. *Economic and Political Weekly*, **12**, 3959-68.

Midanik, L., & Clark, W. (1994). The demographic distribution of US drinking patterns in 1990: description and trends from 1984. *American Journal of Public Health*, **84**, 1218-1222.

Miller, B. (1996). Women's alcohol use and their violent victimization. In Howard, J., Martin, S., Mail, P., Hilton, M., & Taylor, E. (eds.), *Women and alcohol: issues for prevention research*. National Institute on Alcohol Abuse and Alcoholism (NIAAA) Research Monograph No. 32. NIH Publication No. 96-3817. Bethesda, MD: NIAAA, pp. 239-260.

Murthy, N.V., Benegal, V., & Murthy, P. (1995). Alcohol dependent females : a clinical profile, [monograph on the Internet]. Available at http://www.nimhans.kar.nic.in/deaddiction/lit/Female%20Alcoholics.pdf.

Musgrave, S., & Stern, N. (1988). Alcohol demand and taxation under monopoly and oligopoly in South India in the 1970s. *Journal of Development Economics*, **15**, 15-16.

Naik, S. (2002). Indian spirits market: regulatory shackles easing. Mumbai: Rabo India Finance Pvt. Ltd. April 2002, pp. 1-3. Available at: www.rabobank.com/Images/rabobank_publication_indian_spirits_market_2002_tcm25-151.pdf.

Neve, R. J. M., Lemmens, P. H., & Drop, M. J. (1996). Gender differences in alcohol use and alcohol problems: mediation by social roles and gender-role attitudes. *Substance Use Misuse*, **32**, 1439-1459.

Pande, R. *(2000)*. From anti-arrack to total prohibition: the women's movement in Andhra Pradesh, India. *Gender, Technology and Development*, **4**(1), 131-44.

Pittman, D.J. and White, H.R. (eds., 1991). *Society, culture and drinking revisited*. New Brunswick, New Jersey: Rutgers Center of Alcohol Studies.

Plant, M.L. (1997). *Women and Alcohol: Contemporary and Historical Perspectives*, London: Free Association Books.

Plant, M.L., Miller, P., Thornton, C., Plant, M.A., & Bloomfield, K. (2000) Life stage, alcohol consumption patterns, alcohol-related consequences and gender, *Substance Abuse*, **21**, 265-281.

Prasad, S., Murthy, P., Varma, V., Mallika, R., & Gopinath, P.S. (1998). Alcohol dependence in women : a preliminary profile. *NIMHANS Journal*, **16**(1), 87-91

Rahman, L. (2002). Alcohol Prohibition and Addictive Consumption in India [monograph on the Internet]. Available at http://www.nottingham.ac.uk/economics/leverhulme/conferences/postgrad _conf_2003/Rahman_paper.pdf

Rajeswari, R., Chandrasekaran, V., Suhadev, M., Sivasubramaniam, S., Sudha, G., & Renu, G. (2002) Factors associated with patient and health system delays in the diagnosis of tuberculosis in South India. *International Journal of Tuberculosis and Lung Disorders* **6**, 789-795.

Rao, K. N., Begum, S., Venkataramana, V., & Gangadharappa, N. (2001). Nutritional neglect and physical abuse in children of alcoholics. *Indian Journal of Pediatrics* **68**, 843-845.

Ray, S. (2002). Why women get addicted to alcohol. *The Tribune*, Sunday, April 21, 2002, Chandigarh, India. http://www.tribuneindia.com/2002/20020421/herworld.htm

Ray, R., Mondal, A. B., Gupta, K., Chatterjee, A., & Bajaj, P. (2004) The Extent, Pattern and Trends of Drug Abuse in India: National Survey. New Delhi: United Nations Office on Drugs and Crimes & Ministry of Social Justice and Empowerment, Government of India.

Ray, R., & Sharma, H. K. (1994). Drug addiction: an Indian perspective. In V.P. Bashyam (Ed.) *Souvenir of ANCIPS 1994* (pp. 106-109) Madras: Indian Psychiatric Society.

Redgrave, G. W., Swartz, K. L. & Romanoski, A. J. (2003). Alcohol misuse by women. *International Review of Psychiatry*; **15**, 256-268.

Saunders, J.B., Aasland, O.G., Babor, T.F., de la Fuente, J.R., & Grant, M. (1993) Development of the Alcohol Use Disorders Identification Test (AUDIT): WHO collaborative project on early detection of persons with harmful alcohol consumption. II. *Addiction*, **88**, 791-804.

Sarin, S. K., Bhatt, A., Malhotra, V., Sachdev, G., Jiloha, R. C., & Munjal, G. C. (1988). Pattern of alcohol-related liver disease in dependent alcoholics: the Indian dimension. *British Journal of Addiction* **83**, 279-84.

Saxena, S. (1999) Country Profile on Alcohol in India. In : Riley L & Marshall M. (eds) *Alcohol and Public Health in 8 Developing Countries*. Geneva: World Health Organisation . (pp.37-60).

Srinivas, M. N. (1997). Social change in modern India. New Delhi: Orient Longman (p6).

Sri, E. V., Raguram, R., & Srivastava, M.(1997). Alcohol problems in a general hospital—a prevalence study. *Journal of the Indian Medical Association*, **95**, 505-6.

Stockwell, T. (1996). Interventions cannot ignore intentions. *Addiction*, **91**(9), 1283-1284.

Sundaram, K.R., Mohan, D., Advani, G. B., Sharma, H. K., & Bajaj, J. S. (1984)Alcohol abuse in a rural community in India. Part I:Epidemiological Study. *Drug and Alcohol Dependence* **14**, 27–36.

Suresh Kumar, M., & Ray, R. (eds., 2002). *Rapid assessment survey of drug abuse in India* . New Delhi: UNDCP-ROSA and Ministry of Social Justice and Empowerment.

Thimmaiah G (1979) *Socio-economic impact of drinking, State lottery and horse-racing in Karnataka*. New Delhi: Sterling. (pp. 43 & 120).

Wei, H., Derson, Y., Xiao, S., Li, L., & Zhang, Y. (1999) Alcohol consumption and alcohol-related problems: Chinese experience from six area samples, 1994. *Addiction*, **94**(10), 1467-76.

Wilsnack, R.W., & Wilsnack, S.C. (Eds.) *Gender and Alcohol: Individual and Social Perspectives*, New Brunswick, New Jersey: Rutgers Center of Alcohol Studies.

Wilsnack, S. (1996). Patterns and trends in women's drinking: Recent findings and some implications for prevention. In Howard, J., Martin, S., Mail, P., Hilton, M., & Taylor, E. (eds.), *Women and alcohol: issues for prevention research*. National Institute on Alcohol Abuse and Alcoholism (NIAAA) Research Monograph No. 32. NIH Publication No. 96-3817. Bethesda, MD: NIAAA, pp. 19-63.

CHAPTER 6

ALCOHOL CONSUMPTION AMONG MEXICAN WOMEN: IMPLICATIONS IN A SYNCRETIC CULTURE

MARTHA ROMERO MENDOZA, MARIA ELENA MEDINA-MORA,
JORGE VILLATORO & ANA DURAND

INTRODUCTION

Like many other Latin-American countries, Mexico has experienced important social and cultural changes in recent years. At the beginning of the twentieth century the Mexican population consisted of thirteen million inhabitants. During the first three decades the population increased by only three millions, which meant that in 1939 the total number of inhabitants reached sixteen million. During the post revolution period the increase was mainly due to a decrease in mortality. Between 1900 and 1930 the growth rate was 0.7 percent, which in the following two decades reached two percent. In this way, by the middle of the century the Mexican population grew to twenty five millions.

By the year 2000 there were 97 million inhabitants in the country, 48 percent male and 51 percent female (INEGI, 2001). The way the population is distributed in the territory is closely linked with socioeconomic, political, historical, environmental and cultural factors. Of these the most important are the economic growth, the use and availability of resources, infrastructure and services, which determine the conditions of life of the population and their level of wellness. Without a doubt the most important phenomenon that Mexico experienced in the twentieth century was growing urbanization. The human settlement pattern in the country is characterized by a strong concentration of population in a few urban centers and a deep dispersion in small and numerous localities of the country. On the one hand there are cities like the Federal District, the entity with the most population in the country, with more than 5,600 inhabitants per square kilometre; and on the other hand one quarter of the population lives in more than ninety percent of the country, being mostly rural in character and often characterized by poverty and migration. This situation has contributed to changes in the lives of women in Mexico.

THE SITUATION OF WOMEN

It is agreed that no single group of women is a good representation of all women in a particular country. Contemporary women have a diversity of histories, lifestyles and experiences that frame their heterogeneous worlds in relation to language, ecology, available social services, experiences with motherhood or the lack of the latter and the value assigned to this experience in society, violence and of course, health (Lagarde, 1996).

The women's movement for the recognition of their equality with men and the liberation of their sexuality has grown in all the country, with different features and goals but with a deep sense of personal commitment. This movement has transformed the perception women have of their social situation. It affects their every day life, their love relationships, their partners, their relations with others at work, their friends, the way children are raised, and the place of each woman in the social sphere and the cultural production. This change has redefined their roles in love and sex, conditioned their performance with masculine and feminine values in the social sphere and in the life of institutions (Galende, 2001).

Modern Mexican women are syncretic and hybrid. Each one of them reflects the contradictions of two different projects for women's existence. Modernity brings them into contact with universal material and symbolic resources resulting from globalization (Canclini, 1995) while at the same time, each of them has to contend with traditionally established practices. The result of these contradictions is experienced through profound and interminable changes in the nature of their own lives.

According to Canclini (1995), the process of globalization has caused five basic socio-cultural modifications: 1) local and national organizations have lost ground to transnational institutions; 2) the reformulation of the urban environment and the patterns of everyday coexistence (from neighborhoods to condominiums, the workplace, study and activities involving consumption and recreation) are carried out far away from home, limiting the time available to inhabit one's own place; 3) the re-elaboration of identity due to the predominance of goods and messages that come from the global economy and culture; 4) the redefinition of the sense of belonging and identity that is not so much organized through local and national loyalties and more organized through participation in transnational communities (music, fashion, ways of forming couples); and 5) the transition from being a citizen as a representative of public opinion to being a citizen as a consumer interested in enjoying the benefits of a certain way of life.

The tension between these two projects derived from tradition and modernity is simultaneously reflected in two phenomena related to alcohol use: the high rate of female abstainers is paralleled by high rates of hidden consumption, which constitutes a major barrier to treatment.

According to Mexican culture, women are expected to abstain from consuming alcoholic beverages. However, as a result of globalization more women, particularly younger ones with higher educational attainment, are drinking and consequently, some of them are experiencing problems due to this practice. Drinking may be linked to a legitimate right to pleasure (Vance, 1984), yet when women suffer from problems of alcohol abuse or dependence, they do not seek help. When they eventually resort to health services, they have experienced more material and health related losses than men, experienced more rejection from society, their partners have abandoned most of them, and they have experienced more psychological problems.

Women from cultures with a tradition of alcohol use drink and sometimes harm themselves as a result of their drinking. However, the importance of illness is not only related to use. Even women who do not drink are responsible, in their role of mothers, sisters or wives, for preventing alcohol abuse in their significant others. In other words, it is thought that they "can" or "must" control alcohol abuse in their partner, sons or brothers.

In Mexico the consumption of alcohol and other drugs occurs in a context that reflects the way women have been socialized, as well as their status in society. This context affects the way women drink, the type of drinks they choose and how and why they have problems due to their drinking habits. It also affects the resources available for treatment, the barriers they find to asking for help and the effectiveness of the help, if in fact they ever receive it (ARF, 1996).

Very little Mexican research has focused on alcohol use in women (Casco 1993; Medina-Mora, 1993; Romero, 1995; Romero et al, 1997; Romero, 1998). Consequently knowledge in this area has been applied to women on the lack of the consideration of or partial admission that they are different. According to Barret (1990) and Romero (1998), the idea of difference has at least three specific uses: 1) one that effectively records women's situations and experiences; 2) the understanding that its meaning has a positional rather than an absolute nature; and 3) sexual difference.

The aim of this chapter is to present an analysis of the epidemiological data from the National Addiction Survey (NAS) and student surveys, emergency services data related to alcohol use in women, and to reveal the socio-cultural aspects involved in women's alcohol use from a gender perspective.

METHOD

This study uses various methods and possibilities of analysis that provide knowledge on the issue. It combines the results of traditional quantitative methods, such as surveys, with the analysis of a group of in depth interviews and ethnographic observations to obtain an overview of alcohol use in women and at the same time to understand the social construction and significance of these practices.

Data sources

Surveys

The National Addictions Survey (ENA, 1998) is a household survey that was carried out to update information on the prevalence of use of various addictive substances in adults aged 18 to 65. The design of the sample was probabilistic and stratified, with several stages of sampling. A total of 13,228 households were surveyed, from which 12,015 complete interviews were obtained.

The information was gathered through face-to-face interview with a standardized questionnaire containing the basic indicators proposed by the World Health Organization to evaluate substance use/abuse and dependence as well as other problems associated with use. The questionnaires included questions that allowed assessment of use according to socio-demographic variables, social perception of use and risk factors for starting to consume alcohol. The interview took place in a safe and private location and confidentiality was assured.

A total of 43.1% of the interviewees were men and 56.9% were women. The general characteristics of the sample are shown in Table 1. Women in the sample were less educated than men: 6.7% of the women and 3.7% of the males had no formal education. A majority of the sample was Catholic,

TABLE 1.   Demographic characteristics of the sample

Characteristics		Male		Female	
Age	Mean	34.7		34.5	
	SD	12.5		12.1	
		%	n	%	n
Educational Level	None	3.7	89	6.7	222
	Less or equal than 9 years	58.9	1402	65.1	2167
	10 or more years	37.4	891	28.2	940
Religion	Catholic	83.8	1982	86.2	2850
	Protestant or Evangelic	8.9	210	9.7	320
	None	7.3	174	4.1	136
Marital Status	Married	57.2	1361	57.6	1916
	Cohabitating	8.9	211	9.0	301
	Separated/Divorced	2.3	54	6.9	230
	Unmarried	31.1	739	22.6	754
	Widowed	0.6	14	3.8	128
Family Income	Top 25%	18.3	424	14.9	475
	Middle	12.9	299	18.7	594
	Bottom 25%	68.8	1591	66.4	2108
Employment	Involuntary unemployment	99.1	81	2.2	42
	Domestic Work	0.9	1	97.8	1884

married, poor (68.8% of the men and 66.4% of the women had low family income), and most were engaged in domestic work.

In order to determine the interviewees' drinking patterns, they were asked about the frequency with which they consumed various drinks every time they consumed alcohol, as well as the amounts involved. On the basis of this information, 8 different patterns of consumption were determined:

Abstainers: Refers to people who did not consume alcohol during the previous year, whether or not they drank prior to the previous year..

Light, infrequent drinkers: these people reported drinking during the last year, but never more than 5 drinks on any occasion.

Heavy, infrequent drinkers: these people drank during the last year, and sometimes drank 5 or more drinks, but not during the previous month.

*Light, moderately frequent drinker*s: includes those who drank during the previous month but never drank more than 5 or more drinks.

Heavy, moderately frequent drinkers: includes those who drank during the previous month and drank 5 drinks or more on some of these occasions.

Light, frequent drinkers: those who drank during the previous week but never drank more than 5 drinks during the previous year.

Heavy, frequent drinkers: those who drank during the previous week and during the previous year drank 5 or more drinks on some occasions (and did not qualify as heavy, regular drinkers).

Heavy, regular drinkers: those who drank during the previous week and drank 5 or more glasses on one of these occasions.

LIFE HISTORIES

The qualitative data were drawn from the analysis of the life histories of 21 female dependent individuals who voluntarily agreed to participate after receiving information on the project. Each woman was interviewed on at least five occasions, for an hour to an hour and a half. All the semi-structured, open-ended interviews (Hammer and Wildavsky, 1990) were recorded and transcribed literally.

The women who participated in the in-depth interview came from three different contexts: justice institutions (juvenile offenders and women in prison), health institutions for treatment (private and public) and the community (women who were not receiving treatment and women in self-help groups). The women's ages ranged from 14 to 51 years. The analysis was guided by a gender perspective, understood in the way Lagarde (1996) phrased it, as "an analytical methodology that combines various theories linked by their affinity [which] creates a theoretical approach and uses the scientific disciplines of history, anthropology, semiotics, psychology, sociology, economics, political science, aesthetics and philosophy to construct a critical analysis of social subjects" (pp. 45).

RESULTS

PATTERNS OF USE AND CULTURAL NORMS

Cultural expectations are reflected in the social norms that define the rules related to a given practice in a set cultural environment. These rules are specific and determined by status/prestige defined by gender, age, type of occupation, status and positional roles and socio-economic level, among other factors.

Studies conducted in México have shown that nowadays, norms are more concerned with establishing who should drink rather than moderation. Generally speaking, it is thought that women should not drink. Occasional drunkenness among males is regarded as appropriate but among women it is unacceptable, a double standard that is supported by men and women, young and old (Medina-Mora, 1993).

Alcohol consumption in women that does not comply with these standards has traditionally been symbolized as the representation of the transgression of the model of Mexican, occidental, patriarchal femininity. This cultural norm has a dual consequence: if a woman drinks without respecting the limits prescribed for her gender, she will have to conceal or deny her consumption and if she disobeys these norms and is observed by others, she will be strongly rejected and stigmatized (Romero, 1998).

Patterns of consumption in urban women follow these rules, as confirmed by the high rates of abstention. In the 1998 National Addictions survey, 37.7% of the female population had never drunk alcohol, 17.6% admitted to having been former drinkers while only 44.6% of the female population reported being a drinker at the present time.

Table 2 shows the general patterns of consumption of males and females.

In rural and semi-urban villages, this trend is even more pronounced. In a study carried out at the emergency services of three hospitals in Pachuca city, Mexico, 717 women were admitted, 83.9% of whom reported that they were abstainers (Romero et al, 2001).

DEPENDENCE

In the National Addictions Survey (NAS, 1998), 4.6% of the total population ages 18 to 65 met the criteria for the alcohol dependence syndrome. The prevalence for men was 9.6% and 1% for women. Wilsnack (1996) however, has suggested that research on women and alcohol could be improved by measuring and analyzing the wide range of combinations of substances in order to include the synergistic effects of other concurrent drugs. With this in mind, it was decided to analyze the percentage of women dependent on alcohol and drugs. Of the group of women who only consumed alcohol, 1.6% met the criteria for the dependence syndrome, whereas the percentage among those who consumed alcohol and drugs was 3.2%. It is important to note that within the group of symptoms that define

TABLE 2. Drinking patterns by gender and age groups

Frequency of drinking	Males Total %	N	18-29 %	n	30-44 %	n	45-65 %	n	Females Total %	N	18-29 %	n	30-44 %	n	45-65 %	n
Abstainer lifetime	8.7	206	12.3	123	6.5	53	5.4	30	37.7	1256	39.5	538	35.6	442	38.1	276
Ex-Drinker	14.4	344	9.7	97	13	107	25	139	17.6	588	15.9	216	16.7	207	22.7	164
Light infrequent drinker	11.4	272	13.8	138	9.8	81	9.6	54	29.5	982	30	408	31.1	386	26	188
Heavy infrequent drinker	16.3	388	16.6	166	17.5	144	13.9	77	5.1	169	4.5	61	5.6	70	5.2	38
Light moderately frequent drinkers	4.9	118	5.3	53	3.9	32	5.8	32	4.7	156	4.7	64	5.1	63	4	29
Heavy moderately frequent drinkers	18.2	433	17.8	178	22.2	183	13	72	2.6	85	2.6	36	2.7	33	2.2	16
Light frequent drinker	3.6	85	2.8	28	2.4	20	6.6	37	1.4	48	1.4	19	1.5	19	1.3	9
Heavy frequent drinker	6.5	156	5.4	54	7.7	63	7	39	0.6	18	0.6	8	0.9	11	0	0
Heavy regular drinkers	16	381	16.3	163	17.2	142	13.6	76	0.8	27	0.9	12	0.9	11	0.5	4

the dependence syndrome, withdrawal was the most reported symptom.

The percentage of women with the dependence syndrome varied with age, but these results require in-depth study due to the fact that there was no information on the length of time that elapsed between the start of consumption and the time when dependence syndrome began to appear (Figure 1). Likewise, for the group of younger women, it is essential to know when and how they began drinking in this harmful way at such an early age.

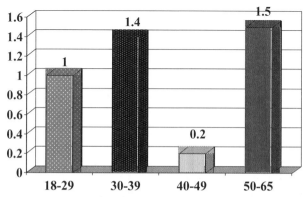

FIGURE 1. Alcohol dependence syndrome by age group

Source: ENA, 1998

TYPE OF DRINKS

A wide range of drinks have been produced in Mexico ever since the time of the conquest. These include fermented drinks, spirits and traditional beverages, such as pulque - a fermented beverage with a low alcohol content obtained from cactus juice, traditionally used in religious and curative rituals by the Aztecs (Berruecos, 1994).

NAS (1998) results show that most women drink beer (28.9%), spirits (23.3%) coolers and table wine (6.6%), and pulque (1.5%). (See Figure 2).

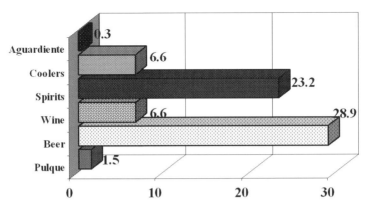

FIGURE 2. Percentage of women drinking different types of beverages

Source: ENA, 1998

YOUTH AND ADVERTISING

There is evidence worldwide that alcohol use among young people begins at increasingly early ages, and that the popularity, variety and availability of low priced alcoholic beverages have increased (Jernigan, 2001).

Young drinkers and women account for a substantial share of the world market and are regarded as key groups for increased consumption. Yoast et al. (1994) estimate that young drinkers who consume alcohol under the legal age constitute 10% of the global market. This emerging group of young consumers tends to prefer beer over wine and spirits (Gabhain and Francois, 2000; Business Research Center, 1997), in addition to a wide range of products with a relatively low alcohol content, such as alcopops, coolers, fortified wines with spirits to raise the alcohol content to 20%, cider and energizing drinks.

Young, single women in Mexico follow this trend. They are able to attend recreational areas that are perhaps unavailable to other women, where they are subjected to social pressure and advertising that encourages them to consume alcohol. In several nightclubs, when couples attend, the women are given drinks at no charge.

A study of 10,578 junior and senior high school students in Mexico City (Villatoro et al, 2000) found that 61.4% of teenagers had consumed alcohol at least once in their lives and that 31.9% had done so during the previous month. An analysis of past month consumption by sex (Figure 3) shows that more men (34%) than women (29%) consume alcohol although the difference is slight. Overall, 60.2% of all women consumed alcohol at some time in their lives, as opposed to 62.6% of men.

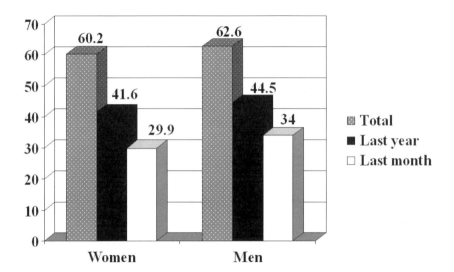

FIGURE 3. Alcohol consumption among Mexican high school students by gender (%; N= 10 578)

Source: Villatoro J, Medina-Mora ME, Blanco J, Villa G, Martínez M, Fleiz C (2000) Encuesta de consumo de drogas en estudiantes. SEP.INPRF II

As for the type of beverage consumed, young women mostly drink five types — beer (44.6%), cocktails (40.2%), spirits (38.4%), wine (26.9%) and canned, blended drinks such as tequila with grapefruit soda or rum and coke (23.6%).

The reasons why young people drink are also split by gender. Whereas women reported drinking alcohol as an emotional escape, when they were experiencing negative emotions, men did so to interact socially and to adapt to situations. (See Figures 4 and 5; Romero et al, 2002).

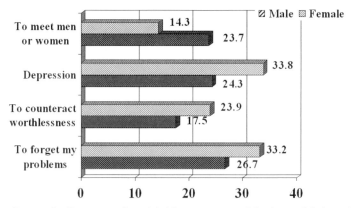

FIGURE 4. Reasons for drinking among Mexican high school students

Source: Romero et al., 2002

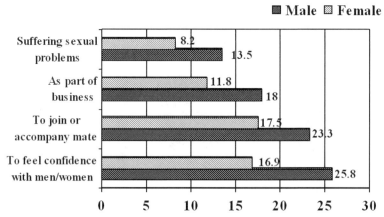

FIGURE 5. Reasons for drinking among Mexican high school students (contd)

Source: Romero et al., 2002

MARITAL STATUS

Factors that influence women's drinking are marital status and partner's drinking patterns, which may modify her pattern of alcohol consumption. Data from the NAS (1998) were analyzed to obtain male and female drinking patterns by demographic characteristics.

Male abstainers tended to be between 45-65 years old, with no formal education, Protestant or evangelical Christian, widowed, with medium income. On the other hand, those males who drank 5 or more drinks per occasion were in the age group of 30-44 years, with the highest educational level, no religious affiliation, separated or divorced and with high income.

Female abstainers were similar to men: they were in the 45-65 age group, with less than or equal to 9 years of school, Protestant, widowed, and with medium income. Females who drank sixty grams or more alcohol per occasion tended to be 30 to 44 years of age, with the highest educational level, cohabitating and with high income.

Romero et al. (2001) found in an emergency service study, that women aged 30 to 49 (55% of the total sample) were most likely to qualify as alcohol abusers. Likewise, women who lived on their own but had had a partner at sometime in their lives (who were separated, divorced or widowed) qualified as alcohol abusers. This was also true for those with higher educational attainment (37.1%). This same study showed that women with harmful consumption of alcohol tended to have partners whose alcohol consumption was moderate or excessive.

Studies conducted in the United States of America yield similar results. In a sample of women aged 24 to 32, Hanna, Faden and Harford (1993) found that alcohol consumption levels decreased in married women or those who had remarried but increased among those who were separated and divorced.

The changes in consumption that accompany a change in marital status may reflect any one of the following hypothesis: 1) a reaction to the imbalance created by instability and a means of adjusting to a new social position; 2) greater autonomy; 3) the fact that the separation was due to the woman's degree of alcohol consumption (Romero, 1999).

VIOLENCE

A recurring problem that has rarely been studied in Mexico is the effect of having been a victim of or observed acts of domestic violence, in other words, having suffered emotional, physical or sexual abuse.

According to a sub-sample of the 1998 National Addiction Survey (NAS), 47% of the total number of women aged 18 to 65 in the urban area living with their partners reported having been victims of violence at some time in their lives, with alcohol being present in 66% of the cases (Observatorio Mexicano, 2002).

Qualitative research shows that this experience is the rule rather than the exception. Women problem drinkers have not only experienced nearly all kinds of violence, but are in a disadvantaged position, since when they lose control, they are thought to be "sexually available", meaning that when they are inebriated, they may be sexually harassed or raped. In some cases, women, especially those that combine alcohol use with other drugs, engage in violent acts, mainly robberies (Romero, 1998).

The main consequences of the link between family violence and excessive alcohol consumption are obviously more serious for women. They often fail to report these incidents out of shame, mainly because of the cultural connotation which regards this behavior as normal, coupled with the uncertainty of how far to put up with this open secret which women suffer in silence. According to Natera (2000) the police and health workers prefer not to "interfere in people's lives". One should not forget the fact that from a gender perspective, "what is personal is political", meaning that violence is both a public health issue and a political problem.

MOTHERHOOD

Expectant women who use alcohol represent many ethical and legal problems, including their reproduction rights, their responsibility for their child's health and the way in which they behave while childrearing. Qualitative research reports that usually the family of origin, legally or illegally, separates the women from their children because of their alcohol consumption. However, one of the main issues in their narratives is their wish to fulfill their role of mothers and their inability to do so, an important source of depression and hopelessness.

> "I drank all the time while pregnant ...when he was born I felt terribly bad...I felt for him rejection...anger...I know that is kind of hard but I wished he died...afterwards he presented seizures and some abnormalities. He was in the emergency service.... After that experience I felt so guilty... I was not married... my mother told me "once a woman is touched by a man it is impossible that you have a partner"... After that I had a suicide attempt... I was in the hospital for two weeks. Up to now if I drink, my brother gets violent with my child...he is two years now... My brother kicks him or put him outside the house in the cold to get me to stop drinking."

> "I became pregnant...and all the time I remembered my mother's words: "If God sends you a child, you have to receive him/her with love like I received you" and at the same time I thought "I will not lose my life by being attached to a baby...all my youth lost...what happens if the baby is born with problems?, without a hand or something?...I decided to have an abortion."

Epidemiological data form the 1989 NAS found that 16% of women drank alcohol during their pregnancy; 8% drank it according to their usual pattern of consumption and 5.7% reduced their alcohol intake; 7.4% of women feeding their last child reported having drunk alcoholic beverages while nursing, especially beer.

Borges et al. (1997) made an in-depth analysis of the NAS women who were pregnant at some time in their lives to study three adverse outcomes during their last pregnancy: spontaneous abortion, stillbirth and congenital abnormalities and their relation to alcohol consumption. Results showed that alcohol consumption during pregnancy was associated with the prevalence of congenital abnormalities, with an odds ratio of 3.4.

MIGRANT WOMEN AND THE INDIGENOUS RURAL POPULATION

In recent decades, the Mexican countryside has been affected by national and global political, economic and social problems that have undermined the structure of traditional peasant production processes as well as the form of social organization. These have influenced their values as well as their individual and collective projects, resulting in increases in alcohol consumption (Berruecos, 2002).

According to Marion (1974), the reconversion of agricultural production has led to greater levels of poverty and an increase in rural-urban migration, which in turn has created rural impoverishment and urban overpopulation. Boltvinik (1995) confirms these data by stating that poverty in Mexico is significantly greater in the countryside than in urban areas, 85% as opposed to 61.7%, according to the National Population Council, with women constituting the most impoverished sector of the population. According to the National Migration Survey (1997) the profile of migrants has been modified by the growing incorporation of rural and urban women into migratory flows.

Oehmichen (20002) states that women who leave their places of origin for the cities do so when they accompany their migrating parents and spouses. Some studies, however, have shown that women's migration is more heavily conditioned than men's by their stage in the life cycle, their position in the household, the presence of children and a partner, and the household structure.

The following are some of the reasons why women leave their communities:

1) The rupture or lack of a bond with a male, either through abandonment or widowhood, in which case the woman assumes responsibility for feeding and looking after the children, if her in-laws and the family of origin lack, the means to support her and her children.

2) For poor indigenous and peasant women, it is one of the few available resources for survival and to a certain extent guaranteeing the survival of their children.

3) Polygyny, understood as a simultaneous marital union between a man and two or more women. This practice often forces second wives to emigrate because they lack the marital status and rights enjoyed by first wives.

4) In association with alcohol consumption, the most important factor for this study. In this case, although a man does not abandon his wife and children, he stops providing for them. Alcohol dependence reduces the financial resources for supporting the family, and also often involves intrafamilial violence, which in turn forces women to migrate.

5) Finally, because of the lack of an acceptable social position for any of several reasons — single motherhood, because the woman already has children or is over the socially acceptable age for marriage, or because the rural community does not provide employment opportunities for her, or a proper marital status.

Patterns of alcohol use in the indigenous cultures display significant variations, providing examples of the complete integration of alcohol use into every aspect of life, as in the case of the Chamula in Chiapas (Polakoff, 2001), or of strict use limited to certain occasions, as among the Tarahumara of Chihuahua.

Among the Chamula, consumption of the traditional beverage called *posh* is a common cause of early death among male drinkers. However, alcohol consumption among women also has serious consequences, as the following paragraph from Polakoff (2001) so poignantly illustrates:

> It took me years to get to the truth. In the past, she had often told me about babies dying as a direct result of the state of inebriation of their mothers, but I would never have imagined the personal event she was referring to. On 9 April 1998, when we were drawing up her family tree, she suddenly told me that a little brother of hers had died on the day he entered the Catholic faith, at the age of about six months, when his mother got drunk during the celebration and dropped him onto the stove. The Chamula authorities put the parents in prison for a few days and I didn't quite know how they got out. She never drinks nowadays, but her friend told me that she didn't stop drinking immediately after the tragedy. She also told me that six out of the original eight children born had died (only she and one of her sisters survived), rather than the three she had originally told me. ´Why didn't you tell me the real number?´ ´Perhaps because I was embarrassed to,´ and we went on writing down the new generations of Chamula (pp. 24-25).

The growth of Protestant religious groups, particularly among rural and indigenous communities, has also had an impact on alcohol consumption patterns and influenced the structure of communities. Indigenous people who have become abstainers after accepting their new religion have had more conflicts with their groups of origin, which have often expelled them from their lands (Díaz-Betancourt, 2004). These conflicts may have numerous origins that warrant in-depth study. For instance, some authors note that these communities reduce the influence of local political bosses in the commercialization of alcohol, thereby affecting their economic interests (Medina-Mora, 1997).

MORTALITY

Mexican women die because of the way they drink. The mortality rate of women aged 15 or over from cirrhosis of the liver caused by drinking has not changed much over the past decade. In 1985, 10.33 out of every 100,000 inhabitants died from this cause, a figure that had risen to 11.20 by 1996 (Medina-Mora, Natera & Borges, 2002)..

In the capital city, the total percentage of deaths related to alcohol consumption in women increased. Data coming from databases recording the forensic causes of death report that in 1999, 10% of female suicides were alcohol-related, a figure that had risen to 25% by 1995. In 1990, 3% of women killed another person when they were inebriated, a figure that had risen to 28.4% by 1995. In 1990, 5.8% of women died in accidents while they were inebriated, and by 1995, this figure had increased to 17.5% (Gutiérrez, 1996).

DISCUSSION

Every woman is involved in the syncretism encapsulated in her person, experiencing the synthesis on the basis of different combinations of depth, complexity and conflict. The syncretic synthesis of identities undergoing a stage of transformation constitutes and organizes the subjectivity of these women who are virtually living double lives. Globalization gives them the opportunity to have access to more public space for leisure but sometimes forces them to migrate because of the economic impact in their communities.

The findings presented in this work should guide reflections on decision making related to public policy regarding prevention, treatment and research specific to women. In the prevention side, intervention strategies should be specifically designed for women, and treatment should focus attention on the medical and psychosocial needs of dependent women. Finally, more effort should be made to overcome treatment barriers and prejudices against women with alcohol-related problems.

REFERENCES

Addiction Research Foundation (1996). *The hidden majority. A guidebook on alcohol and other drug issues for counselors who work with women.* Toronto: Addiction Research Foundation.

Barret, M. (1990). El concepto de diferencia.[The concept of difference] *Debate feminista*. September, 311-325.

Berruecos, L. (1994). Bebidas y Licores de Hoy [Today's beverages and liquors]. In: *Bebidas Nacionales. Guía México Desconocido* [Nacional Beverages. Unknown Mexico Guide] .No.18, Editorial Jilguero, S.A. de C.V. Mexico City: Noviembre.

Berruecos, L. (2003). La transformación de los patrones de consumo de alcohol, como resultado de la globalización, en una zona indígena de México.[The transformation of alcohol consumption patterns as a result of globalization, in an indigeneous zone of Mexico]. *Perspectivas Políticas,* **16**, 1-34.

Boltvinik, J. (1995). La pobreza en México.[Poverty in Mexico] *Salud Pública de México,* **1**(37), 298-309.

Bordieu, P., & Waquant, L. (1995). *Respuestas. Por una antropología reflexiva.* [Responses. For a reflexive anthropology] Mexico City: Grijalbo.

Borges, G., Tapia-Conyer, R., López-Cervantes, M., Medina-Mora, M. E., Pelcastre, B., & Franco, F. (1997). Alcohol consumption and pregnancy in the Mexican national addiction survey. *Caderno Saude Publica,* **13** (2), 205-211.

Canclini, N. (1995). *Consumidores y ciudadanos. Conflictos multiculturales de la globalización.* [Consumers and citizens. Multicultural conflicts in the globalization] Mexico City: Grijalbo.

Casco, M., Natera, G. (1993). El alcoholismo en la mujer: la explicación que ellas mismas dan. [Alcoholism in women: the explanation they give] *Salud Mental,* **16**(1), 24-29.

Díaz-Betancourt, J. (2004). Huicholes católicos expulsan de su comunidad a evangélicos. [Catholic huicholes expelled from their community to evangelics] Agenda, Martes 10 de Febrero, *La Jornada*, México.

ENA (1998). Encuesta Nacional de Adicciones.[National Survey on Addictions] Ed. Subsecretaría de Prevención y Control de Enfermedades. Dirección General de Epidemiología. Instituto Mexicano de Psiquiatría. Consejo Nacional contra las Adicciones. Mexico City: Secretaría de Salud.

Galende, E (2001). Sexo y Amor. Anhelos e incertidumbres de la intimidad actual. [Sex and love. Uncertainties and wishes of the actual intimacy]. Buenos Aires: Paidós.

Gutiérrez, R. (1996). Bases de datos sobre estadísticas de alcohol.[Databases on alcohol statistics] Mexico City, Mexico: Centro de Información sobre alcohol. Instituto Mexicano de Psiquiatría,.

Hammer, D., Wildavsky, A. (1990). La entrevista semi-estructurada de final abierto. Aproximación a una guía operativa. [The open-ended semi-structured interview] *Historia y Fuente Oral,* **4**, 23-61.

Hanna, E., Faden, V,, Harford, T. H, (1993). Marriage: does it protect young women from alcoholism? *Journal of Substance Abuse,* **5** (1),1-14.

INEGI (2001). Indicadores sociodemográficos de México [Sociodemographic numbers of México] México City, Mexico: Ed. Instituto Nacional de Estadística, Geografía e Informática.

Jeringan, D. (2001). Alcohol and young people. Global Status Report. Mental Health and Substances Dependence Department. Geneva: World Health Organization.

Lagarde, M. (2001). Identidad Femenina.[Feminine Identity] CIDHAL, Lecturas y Noticias. http:/www.laneta.apc.org/cidhal/lectura/identidad/texto3.htm.

Lagarde, M. (1996). *Género y feminismo. Desarrollo humano y democracia.* [Gender and feminism. Human development and democracy] Madrid: Ed. Horas y horas. Cuadernos inacabados. Número 25.

Marion, M. (1995). El derecho de pensar diferente.[The right of thinking different] *Psiquiatría.* Época 2, **11**(2), 52-55.

Medina-Mora, M. E. (1993). Diferencias por género en las prácticas de consumo de alcohol. [Gender differences in alcohol consumption practices] Tesis para la obtención de grado de doctora en Psicología Social. Mexico City, Mexico: Facultad de Psicología. UNAM.

Medina-Mora, M, E. (1997). Alcohol policies in developing countries. Mexican report. Paper presented for the alcohol policies in developing countries meeting. Mexico, City, April.

Medina-Mora, M. E., Natera, G., Borges, G. (2002). Alcoholismo y abuso de bebidas alcohólicas.[Alcoholism and abuse of alcoholic beverages] En: *Observatorio Mexicano en tabaco, alcohol y otras drogas*. México City, Mexico: Ed. Consejo Nacional contra las Adicciones..

Natera, G., López, J. L., Tiburcio, M., Martín-Barba, R. M., & León Pérez, J. (2000). Violencia y alcohol, una relación peligrosa.[Violence and alcohol, a dangerous relationship] En: Viveros M. *Niñez, Adolescencia y Género, una propuesta desde la educación y la salud por la no violencia*.[Adolescence and gender, a propoasal from the education and health for no violence]. México City, Mexico: Fundación Mexicana para la Salud.

Observatorio Mexicano en tabaco, alcohol y otras drogas (2002). Violencia familiar y consumo de alcohol.[Domestic violence and alcohol consumption] Revisión bibliográfica. Mexico City, Mexico: Ed. Consejo Nacional contra las Adicciones.

Oehmichen, C. (2000). Las mujeres indígenas migrantes en la comunidad extraterritorial. [The migrant indigenous women in the extraterritorial community]. In: Barrera D, Oehmichen C: *Migración y relaciones de género en México*. [Migration and gender relations in Mexico] Mexico City, Mexico: Ed. GIMTRAP e Instituto de Investigaciones Antropológicas, UNAM..

Polakoff, K. (2001). Del trago a la tragedia: el consumo de alcohol en San Juan Chamula, Chiapas. [From swig to tragedy: alcohol consumption in San Juan Chamula, Chiapas]. Tesis para obtener el grado de maestra en antropología. Instituto de Investigaciones Antropológicas. Mexico City, Mexico: Facultad de Filosofía y Letras, UNAM.

Romero, M. (1995). Sobre la necesidad de conceptuar el género en el estudio de las adicciones. [On the need of conceptualizing gender in addictions studies] *Psicología y Salud*. Instituto de Investigaciones Psicológicas de la Universidad Veracruzana. 5 Enero-Junio, 135-146.

Romero, M. (1998). Estudio de las adicciones a sustancias psicoactivas en mujeres y su relación con otros problemas de salud mental. [Study on women's addiction and its relationship with other mental health problems].Tesis de doctorado en antropología. Instituto de Investigaciones Antropológicas. Facultad de Filosofía y Letras. UNAM.

Romero, M. (1999). Diversidad femenina y consumo de alcohol.[Feminine diversity and alcohol consumption] In: La mujer en la cultura del consumo de bebidas con alcohol: riesgos y beneficios". *Cuadernos FISAC,* **1** (3)**,** 47-61.

Romero, M., Gómez, C., Ramiro, M., & Díaz, A. (1997). Necesidades de atención a la salud mental de la mujer adicta.[Mental Health attention needs of addicted women] *Salud Mental,* **20**(2), 38-47.

Romero, M., Mondragón, L., Cherpitel, S., Medina-Mora, M. E., & Borges, G. (2001). Characteristics of Mexican women admitted to emergency care units. Alcohol consumption and related problems. *Salud Pública de México* **43**(6), 537-543.

Romero, M., Villatoro, J., Fleis, C., Medina-Mora, M. E. (2002). Gender differences in reasons for drinking: results of a Mexican Student Survey. Paper presented at the Kettil Brunn Society Symposium, Paris.

United Nations, UNDCP, WHO (1994) Subcommittee on Drug Control. *Women and Drug Abuse. A positional paper.* Geneva: WHO.

Vance, C. (1984). Pleasure and danger: towards a politics of sexuality. In Vance, C., *Pleasure and danger: exploring female sexuality.* London: Routledge & Kegan.

Villatoro, J., Medina-Mora, M. E., Rojano, C., Fleiz, C., Villa, G., Jasso, A., Alcàntar, M., Bermúdez, P., Castro, P., Blanco, J. (2001). *Consumo de drogas, alcohol y tabaco en estudiantes del Distrito Federal: Medición otoño 2000.* [Drugs, alcohol and tobacco consumption in students from the Federal District: Autumn report 2000] Reporte Global del Distrito Federal, INP-SEP, México.

Yoast, R., Larkin, L., Sherman, J. (2001). *Partner or foe? The alcohol industry, youth alcohol problems and alcohol policy strategies. Policy briefing paper.* Alcohol issues. Chicago: American Medical Association.

Wilsnack, S. (1996). Patterns and trends in women's drinking: recent findings and some implications for prevention. In J. Howard, M. Marin, M. Hilton (eds.), *Women and Alcohol: issues for prevention research* (pp. 19-63). Rockville, MD: US National Institute on Alcoholism and Alcohol Abuse (NIAAA) Research Monograph 32.

CHAPTER 7

THE CONTEXTS OF ALCOHOL CONSUMPTION IN NIGERIA

AKANIDOMO J. IBANGA, ADEBOLA V. ADETULA, ZUBAIRU DAGONA,
HARUNA KARICK & OCHIYNA OJIJI

INTRODUCTION

Nigeria is easily one of the most diverse and complex polities on the African continent. It is distinguished from most other developing countries by its population of approximately 135 million people, with high concentration of youths below the age of 20 years. Nigeria gained political independence from Britain in 1960. However, in its nearly 50 years of independence Nigeria has often been under military rule.

The long period of military rule had, to a certain degree, a negative impact on the development of the country. Although Nigeria returned to civil rule in May 1999, the new government's promise of macro-economic policy reform, poverty alleviation, improved service delivery, universal basic education, accountability of government and reduced corruption, is yet to be realized. The economy is relatively stagnant, growing in 2002 at a rate of just 3.3%, less than half what is required to reduce poverty, and only slightly higher than the annual population growth rate of 2.8%. Per capital income is just $300 per year; 70% of Nigerians live in poverty on less than $1 per day, and at least 15% of Nigerian children die before reaching their fifth birthday. The country has low adult literacy rate of 58 % for men, and 41 % for women. The population growth rate is high, and the population is expected to reach 270 million in less than 25 years. The overall development environment in Nigeria is captured in the United Nations Development Programme Human Development Index which ranks Nigeria 151st out of 177 countries (UNDP, 2002).

During the economic boom of the 1970s, the country recorded rapid economic development and experienced one of the fastest urbanization rates in the world. However, poor leadership style and mismanagement of the oil boom of the 1970s resulted in a serious economic downturn in the 1980s. The estimates of the urban growth rate in 1970 -1980 ranged from 16 to 27%. In 1995 it was estimated to be 40%. Rural-urban migration increased with the development of urban centres; adolescents and particularly young adult males, migrated in their thousands from the rural areas to urban centres in search of jobs. This movement, largely compelled by economic forces, may add to distress and the anomie that can enhance the attractions of drinking and drunkenness, and may remove some of the cultural constraints on alcohol consumption and subsequent behaviour such as violence. Thus urbanization and employment-induced mobility, and in recent times, mobility induced by the sporadic ethnic and religious crises within the country, puts the stability of the Nigerian family in some jeopardy, a factor that has been associated with drug use (Ndom & Adelekan, 1996). Other consequences of the rural-urban drift include a decrease in agricultural productivity, and a decline in the influence of the extended family and community, as well as increased salience of the peer group. This pattern seems similar to those of many industrialized countries where deficiencies in social support have made young people more vulnerable to the urban environment (Ferguson, 1993). Rapid urbanization and social dislocation have been linked with increased consumption of alcohol in Nigeria (Ebie & Pela, 1981; Lambo, 1965), especially in the 1960s and 1970s when the abuse of alcohol became quite prominent in the country.

HISTORY OF ALCOHOL CONSUMPTION IN NIGERIA

Alcohol consumption has a long history in Nigeria, and its use is common in all the cultural groups in the country. It is one of the most available psychoactive substances in the country, and it is consumed either in the form of traditional beverages (e.g., *burukutu, pito, emu funfun,* palm-wine, *ogogoro*), or as western lager beer, wine or spirituous liquors (e.g., brandy, whisky and gin). In many parts of the country, the production and consumption of alcoholic beverages was organized around traditional rituals, festivals and other social activities which included arrangements around marriages, childbearing and child-naming, weekly market days, and settling of quarrels between families and communities. Presenting or offering alcoholic beverage was also an expression of hospitality to visiting guests.

The works of Netting (1964) and Odejide & Olatuwura (1977) have shown that in some cultures, the use of alcohol, especially by social groups during festivals and ceremonies, is usually associated with rituals to highlight the hierarchies within a particular social group or community. This may take the form of passing the traditional wine cup around in a gathering in a particular order that gives primacy to age and title (Umana, 1967). While the age groups of men and women were often not explicitly separated during these occasions, elders and men were expected to drink more than either young men or women (Oshodin, 1995).

In traditional Nigerian society, daily consumption of alcoholic beverages was not the norm, as drinking revolved around festivals, rituals and important ceremonies. Additionally, these occasions allowed for the exercise of control over who is served or not served, and the quantity which they are served. In this way people were somewhat protected from drinking excessively. This is evident in some expressions of culturally constructed norms that decry excessive drinking. It was however possible that outside these circumscribed settings, alcohol was produced and used privately. When consumed in this way it could be in excess of culturally permitted limits and could result in intoxication (Obot, 1993a). It was not so much that excessive drinking was not tolerated, but becoming intoxicated by drinking was looked down on and incurred sanctions. On the other hand, being able to drink large quantities without noticeable evidence of intoxication was considered admirable (Gureje et al., 1996).

The point being made here is that in traditional Nigerian societies the widespread consumption of large quantities of alcohol was relatively uncommon. It can be said that abuse of alcohol became prominent in the 1960s and 1970s, with the increased and widespread use of western alcoholic beverages. In earlier centuries western alcoholic beverages were introduced into Nigeria by explorers, who initially brought them as gifts for African chiefs. Later on, especially during the transatlantic slave trade, these alcoholic beverages were part of the articles of trade used in exchange for slaves and other exports from the West African coast. This was the foundation for the eventual introduction of alcohol as a commercial product in modern international trade between Nigeria and Europe. During the colonial era these beverages (introduced initially by the explorers) usually had higher alcohol content than the local beverages, and were soon considered socially harmful commodities by the colonial authorities.

TYPES OF TRADITIONAL ALCOHOLIC BEVERAGES

Alcoholic beverages featured prominently in many traditional Nigerian cultural groups. Traditional alcoholic beverages were processed from local raw materials by methods handed down from previous generations. In the North central parts of Nigeria, the common alcoholic beverages are *burukutu* and *pito* produced from grains (maize, millet , or guinea corn). The production of *burukutu* and *pito* is labour intensive and it is mostly carried out by women. Another local alcoholic beverage peculiar to the southern parts of the country is palmwine. Palmwine is tapped from the raffia and oil palm trees and it remains a popular drink. A distillate of palmwine—a spirit with high alcohol content—known locally as *akpetesh, kinkana, fire water or ogogoro* is also available and consumed all over the country.

The historical significance of *ogogoro* lies in the fact that it was banned by the British administrators as part of attempts to control the West African liquor trade. Because it was considered an illicit gin, its production went underground, but was never really halted. In response to the desires of the people the independent national government in 1970 lifted the ban on its production and sale.

THE ALCOHOL INDUSTRY

The production and distribution of alcohol is handled by people in both formal and informal sectors of the Nigerian economy. The informal sector is largely unregulated, with little or no government control. This is more evident in regards to domestically produced alcoholic beverages. For the most part, alcoholic beverages are easily available in many makeshift, street-corner kiosks in both rural and urban centres. The government, thus, does not have accurate records of quantities produced, or the retail outlets for these beverages. Cultural and religious restrictions, in some instances, may confine the production, distribution, sale and the consumption to certain areas of the cities.

The formally organized liquor industry in Nigeria has developed into a sector dominated by two main companies: Nigerian Breweries Plc and Guinness Nigeria Plc. They are reportedly the two largest capitalized companies on the Nigerian Stock Exchange (Uzor, 1999). As noted by Obot, Ibanga and Karick (2002) in a review of the history of beer production in Nigeria, Nigerian Breweries Plc., though established in 1945, produced the first bottle of beer on the 14th July 1949. It was also within this period that a company was formed to import Guinness Extra Stout into the country from Ireland. The increasing demand for the product led to the establishment of a Guinness brewery in 1962. This was the third Guinness brewery worldwide and the first ever to be established outside of Ireland and the United Kingdom. Today, there are three Guinness breweries in the country. Guinness stout is sold in both 30cl and 60cl bottles. Lager beer, on the other hand, is produced and sold in 60cl bottles, approximately twice the size of a typical beer container in western countries. The Standard Organization of Nigeria specifies a minimum of 3% ethanol content for lager and 6% for stout. A typical beer contains about 4%.

The success of these two alcohol enterprises led to establishment of more breweries. In 1979 there were 9 breweries, this grew to 34 by 1982, among them producing more than 40 brands of beer. Of the 34 breweries, 27 (80%) were situated in the southern parts of the country and only 7 (20%) were in the north. Along with these breweries were four distilleries and nine wineries (Federal Office of Statistics, 1985). The location of these industries may in part be a reflection of the demand pattern and the differential attitudes towards the use of alcohol between the northern and the southern parts of Nigeria. On the other hand, it may be as a result of polarization in the country brought about by the differential application of the enactment of the Liquor Amendment Ordinance No. 26 of 1919, as suggested by Gureje (1999). The enactment of this ordinance put the whole northern part of Nigeria under a different set of rules in regards to alcohol use than the southern parts. It is important to note that northern Nigeria is predominantly Muslim while the south is predominantly Christian.

The economic downturn in the 1980s came with the devaluation of the currency and the scarcity of foreign exchange for imported inputs. The

Nigerian government compelled the industry to substitute local raw materials for the imported ones. The resulting investment in plant and machinery necessary to convert production lines to handle local raw materials, and the dwindling purchasing power of the general populace experiencing economic recession, combined to kill some of the breweries. Most hit were the regional brands that were owned by state governments; about 3 out of every 4 of these plants disappeared from the scene by 1996. The two dominant players in the alcohol industry, however, consolidated their position. The volume of beer produced in the country did show an increase between 1984 and 1994. The domestic production of beer rose from 7,354.7 million hectolitres in 1984 to 23,970.1 million hectolitres in 1994 (Federal Office of Statistics, 1995; Akerele, 1993). This volume is still well below the installed capacity.

As we have noted earlier, the brewing industry in Nigeria is a very profitable one. The reports of the Federal Office of Statistics show that even though aggregate index of industrial production in the country fell in 1993 by 3.1%, with manufacturing declining by 4.1%, the brewing industry actually grew by about 8.5% in the same period. This growth had a spill-over effect particularly in the communities where these companies were situated. Switching to the use of local raw materials as a result of the earlier ban on foreign raw materials led to a boost in local agriculture. The beer companies created jobs which allowed for employment of large numbers of people both directly and indirectly. For many in localities where the industries are sited, the beer trade became the primary economic activity. It contributed specifically towards raising the economic profile of women who constitute the greater proportion of retailers.

The existing breweries seem to have recovered from this switch and are today making profits in comparison to other industries that are downsizing. The Nigeria Brewery Plc, for instance, had a turnover that jumped from 17.7 billion naira in 2000 to 29.7 billion in 2001 (about USD $220 million at exchange rates in 2005). Profit before tax was up from 6.5 billion naira to 10 billion in the years under consideration. Its share price of 25.50 naira in December 2000 rose to 57.00 naira by the first half of 2002.

ALCOHOL MARKETING AND PROMOTION IN NIGERIA

Marketing and promotion of alcoholic beverages has largely been unrestrained in Nigeria. The emergence of democracy and the liberalization program of the government have both attracted a flow of capital into different sectors of the economy, as well as opening the Nigerian market to all types of imported alcoholic beverages. The removal of excise duty in 1998 helped the sector to cut prices, increase turnover and enhance profit. Alcohol brewers have also become more aggressive in their advertising, making use of the radio, television, billboards and print media. The common theme in these advertisements is that drinking is a fun, modern and enlightening activity; it brings friends together; it is for the successful and comes with prestige. Usually the scenes depict young and upwardly mobile men pictured alongside women having fun. The impact of this form of advertisement is seen in the image of drinking as a substitute for other forms of recreation (Gureje et al., 1996). Adverts have also tried to capture the distinct nature and/or "good quality" of the particular alcoholic beverages (Obot & Ibanga, 2003; Obot, Ibanga & Karick, 2002).

In the recent past, the brewing industry has adopted marketing and promotion strategies that target particular sections of the Nigerian populace. Some of the strategies adopted include sponsoring of essay competitions at all levels, fashion shows, sports events, musical segments, end of year carnivals, radio call-in shows, lottery type free drinks, and discounted drinks, in-bar promotion, and "fun fare" where alcoholic beverages are offered free. In this way the alcohol industry aims to worm its way into the lives of people in the society.

DRINKING PATTERNS

Initial research on alcohol and drug use was initiated as a result of casual observations that a significant number of young people were being admitted into psychiatric hospitals because of abuse of drugs, particularly cannabis and alcohol (Asuni, 1964; Lambo, 1965). Clinical studies conducted in psychiatric facilities in Nigeria found drug-related admission accounted for up to 11% of all admissions. In all these studies (Ahmed, 1986; Obot & Olaniyi, 1991; Ikwuagu et al., 1993; 1989; Ohaeri & Odejide, 1993) cannabis contributed most to drug-related problems, followed by alcohol. Only in one study (Ahmed, 1986) was alcohol more commonly abused than other drugs, as determined by admission records in the psychiatric hospital over a five-year period.

Surveys among students in secondary schools and tertiary institutions have been conducted over the years. Despite the limitations in epidemiological studies conducted in the country (Obot, 1993b; Ibanga, 1997; Obot et al., 2001) there is evidence on the extent of drug use among students. Anumoye (1980), in a survey of 17 secondary schools, reported that 20% had taken alcohol at least once. In the ICAA (1988) surveys in southern Nigeria the proportion of students who had ever used alcohol ranged from 24.4% to 49.2%. Higher rates ranging from 56% - 79% have been found (Oshodin, 1981; Nevadomsky, 1982; Idowu, 1987; Odejide et al., 1987; Obot, 1999).

Apart from these independent studies, the National Drug Law Enforcement Agency (NDLEA) has conducted several surveys of drug and alcohol use among secondary school students in different parts of the country (NDLEA, 1992, 1993, 2000). Results of the studies showed a clear difference in the use of alcohol in the north and south of the country. The rates of drinking reported among the youths in the northern city (Kano) were much lower than the rates reported by students in the southern city of Lagos. This difference could be attributed to religion, the north being predominantly Muslim while most southerners are Christians. Equally high rates have been recorded for out-of-school youths (Obot, 2001).

In tertiary institutions the rates of drinking are slightly higher. Oladimeji and Fabiyi (1993) reported past year use of alcohol as 66.4% and 84%, respectively, in 1984 and 1988. Oshodin (1982) found that 87% of the males and 79% of the females had drunk alcohol in their lifetime; 78% of them had started drinking before entry into colleges, and 71% had increased their drinking.

A few general population surveys have been conducted in Nigeria. Three surveys conducted in different parts of the country fit into this category. The first is the ICAA study of drug abuse in the southern parts of the country. Second was the study of drinking behaviour conducted among civil servants to determine the pattern of psychotropic drug use (a study among civil servants is not a general population survey). In a sample of 5,320 literate civil servants they found that beer was consumed by 45.7% of the respondents, wine by 43.2 %, and spirits by 32.8%. Lastly, Obot (1993) conducted a general population survey in the North Central region of the country. Data on drinking and alcohol use was collected from 1,052 heads of households; 52.5% of the sample described themselves as alcohol drinkers. A high proportion of them (39.2%) drank some form of alcohol at least once a day, and many of them showed a pattern of heavy consumption of alcoholic beverages.

ALCOHOL-RELATED PROBLEMS

In traditional Nigerian culture male social drinking is approved but attracts social sanctions. Women's drinking was determined, however, by the quantity they were allowed by men to take on certain occasions. Since these controls are no longer in force, more uncontrolled drinking occurs in both sexes, which might result in an increasing prevalence of alcohol-related problems. The absence of detailed records in most hospitals makes accurate estimates of alcohol-related morbidity difficult. Only a few hospitals keep records that would allow for the determination of such disorders as liver cirrhoses or pancreatitis, thus allowing a full determination of the contribution of alcohol to health problems.

Surveys in primary care facilities show that a significant number of those attending these clinics for diverse medical problems, especially males, would have evidence of ICD-9 or DSM-IIIR diagnosis of alcohol abuse or dependence (Ifabumuyi, 1982; Guruje et al., 1992, 1995). Findings from the ICAA (1988) study point to the fact that a disproportionate part of total admissions in tertiary hospital beds is linked to alcohol misuse. At the level of social functioning, problem drinkers have been shown to experience more problems than non-heavy drinkers. They experience more accidents, violence, disruption of family, work, and social relationships (Ibanga, 1998, 2002; Obembe, 1988; Obot 1993, 2001; Obot & Obot, 1995).

CURRENT RESPONSE

The rising drug problem in the country in the 1980s and 1990s placed Nigeria in a negative light internationally. In response to this, the government established the National Drug Law Enforcement Agency (NDLEA), an agency that focuses largely on the control of supply and reduction of demand for illicit substances. The Government has made strides in the direction of interdiction and enforcement of law regarding production and trafficking. The consideration of issues of abuse of licit drugs, however, has not received such attention or public outcry. For instance, though laws exist with respect to production, distribution and consumption of alcoholic beverages, the government has not enforced such laws and the public is to a large extent ignorant of their existence. The non-enforcement of these laws could be in part due to the immense benefit that the government derives in the form of tax from the alcohol industry. It may also be out of the recognition that alcohol is an integral part of the daily and ceremonial life of many Nigerians. Compared with many other countries, the Nigerian government is not strict in implementing policies that regulate alcohol production, distribution and consumption.

As this review points out, much still remains to be known about alcohol consumption in Nigeria. There has been no general population study that takes an in-depth look at the situational context in which alcohol consumption occurs. The present study was designed to address this issue by taking into account possible factors that may be associated with consumption in the different situations. This study assessed the extent of alcohol consumption in the general population of Nigerian and provides an insight into gender differences in the types of alcoholic beverages consumed and the frequency of drinking of alcoholic beverages in different contexts.

METHOD

SAMPLE

The sample was drawn from two out of the six political zones in the country: one in the north and the other in the south. Three states and the Federal Capital Territory were selected in the north (Benue, Nasarawa, Plateu), and two states in the south (Akwa Ibom, Rivers). Each state had 60 enumeration areas that had been mapped out and listed. Of the 60 enumeration areas (EA) in each state, 40 were chosen randomly. Where the household unit contained more than one housing unit, the housing unit used was selected using a table of random numbers. Ultimately ten household units were selected from each of the 40 EAs for inclusion in the survey. In these household units one adult member of the household was designated as the respondent from a table of random numbers. The selected adult was between the ages of 18 and 65 years. Excluded from the sample were people who were institutionalized, hospitalized, in school, or had no official residence as at the time of the survey.

Thus there were 400 respondents in each of the five states sampled. Since the Federal Capital Territory has a smaller population than the states, a total of 20 out of 30 enumeration areas were sampled. In this case 15 housing units were selected from each enumeration area, thus giving a total of 300 respondents. Consequently the total number of respondents expected in the sample was 2,300. Representativeness was achieved through the selection of respondents based on other variables like sex and age. Because of the need to sample relatively equal number of males and females, each interviewer alternated from house-to-house between the males and females in the choice of the adult member to interview. Sampling thus involved a number of stages. The first stage was the selection of the enumeration areas. The second stage involved sampling the households that were listed. The third stage involved sampling of housing units where there was more than one housing unit in a household (address). The final stage involved selecting the individuals within the housing unit. Data collection took place between October and November 2002.

PROCEDURE

Male and female interviewers were recruited from the Federal Office of Statistics, and trained for the purpose of this study. The interviewers were trained in two separate locations for the separate regions of the country. This training was done by members of the research planning team and consultants.

Actual data collection from some of the areas posed a challenge. Due to the terrain in some states, interviewers had to travel by diverse means (bicycle or boat) to access some of the chosen enumeration areas. In some areas of Plateau State, for instance, there were outbreaks of communal violence at the time of the survey which made access to those communities somewhat difficult. In these areas interviewers had to wait for days before data collection could proceed. Most of the refusals that would have come from community heads in these situations were averted as the interviewers were known for their data collecting roles for the Federal Office of Statistics in the past.

MEASURES

The questionnaire used in this study was a slightly modified version of the questionnaire designed by International Research Group on Gender and Alcohol (IRGGA). It was a highly structured questionnaire with defined response codes. It consisted of more 300 questions divided into 9 different sections: demographics, work experience, social networks, drinking variables, familial and other drinking context, drinking consequences, intimate relations and sexuality, violence/victimization, health and life style. Patterns of alcohol consumption were based on respondents' self-report of the frequency during the past 12 months that they drank any kind of alcoholic beverage as well as the quantity of alcohol they took on a typical day that they drank.

DRINKING FREQUENCY

Frequency of taking specific alcoholic beverages was also assessed with the number of drinks that the individual consumes on a typical day. The response categories for the questions on frequency were:

> Every day or nearly every day, Three or four times a week, Once or twice a week, One to three times a month, Seven to eleven times in the last 12 months, Three to six times in the last 12 months, Twice in the last 12 months, Once in the last 12 months, or Never in the last 12 months.

For the analysis these options were recoded into five categories as follows.

> Daily or nearly daily, Weekly, Monthly, Less than monthly, Never in the last 12 months.

The quantity of drinks they consumed was obtained by asking the respondents to report the number of drinks they had on a typical day they were drinking. This was assessed for alcoholic beverages in general as well as for each type alcoholic beverages.

Abstainers were required to answer questions about their experience with alcohol. Those who had never drunk any beverage containing alcohol in their lives were lifetime abstainers; those who had not had a drink within the past 12 months were current abstainers. These were asked to provide reasons for not drinking by responding "yes" or "no" to 16 possible reasons including, lack of interest , cost, taking medication, religion and disliking the taste.

CONTEXT OF DRINKING

Questions were asked of all drinkers to examine the frequency of drinking in different contexts within the last 12 months. Respondents were required to state how much drinking occurred in the following contexts:

> During mealtime, At a party or celebration, In own home, At friend's home, At workplace, In a bar, In a restaurant

The response categories were:

> Every day or nearly every day, Three or four times a week, Once or twice a week, One to three times a month, Seven to eleven times in the last 12 months, Three to six times in the last 12 months, Once or twice in the last 12 months, Never in the last 12 months.

These responses were recoded to: *Weekly or more, Monthly, Less than monthly, Never in the last 12 months.*

Apart from gender, the demographic characteristics assessed in the survey and used in the present analysis were age, education, and area of residence. Age was recoded as: *18–29 years, 30–44 years, 45+ years.* Education was recoded into the following categories: *No formal education, 1–9 year, > 9 years.*

Area of residence was classified as rural and urban, based on criteria used by the Federal Office of Statistics.

RESULTS

CONSUMPTION PATTERNS

Table 1 shows drinking by selected demographic variables. Drinking was generally a male behaviour with 41.5% being current drinkers, as opposed to 22% among the females in this survey. This difference was

TABLE 1. Percentages of respondents reporting consumption of alcoholic beverage in the past year by selected socio-demographic characteristics

Socio-demographic characteristics	n	Current drinker (%)
Total sample	2099	32.5
Gender**		
Male	1126	41.5
Female	958	22.0
Educational level*		
No formal education	779	28.6
1-9 Years	1040	35.2
10+ years	249	32.9
Residence**		
Urban	788	27.4
Rural	1281	35.5
Marital status		
Married	1474	32.4
Cohabiting	46	23.9
Widowed	121	35.5
Divorced	24	50.0
Married but separate	35	48.6
Single	371	30.2
Age**		
18-29 Years	603	21.1
30-44 Years	821	34.8
45+ Years	611	40.9
Religion**		
Christian	1735	36.1
Muslim	297	8.8
Other	32	50.0
Household income*		
Low	1555	33.1
Middle	292	38.4
High	191	23.0

* $p< 0.01$
** $p<0.001$
Note: Percentages are based on the number of valid responses.

found to be statistically significant (x^2 =91.05, $p<0.001$). Overall, the highest proportion of drinkers (40 %) fell within the age bracket of 45 years and above and the least was among respondents who were between the ages of 18–29 years (21.1%). In regards to religion, those adhering to traditional African religion were much more likely to be current drinkers (50%) than Christians (36.1%). Muslims were significantly less often current drinkers (8.8%). The difference among the religious groups was also found to be statistically significant (x^2 = 91.01, $p<0.001$).

With respect to marital status, those who were cohabiting, single or married (23.9%, 30.2%, and 32.4%, respectively) had lower rates for alcohol consumption than those who were widowed (35.5%). The higher proportions of alcohol consumption were found in the divorced and separated groups (50% and 48.6% respectively). Cross-tabulations of marital status and heavy drinking (5 or more drinks on a typical drinking occasion) were also obtained. The results showed that 82.4% of those who were married but separated drank heavily, followed by the divorced (58.3%), and the married (52.6%). Those that were cohabiting had the lowest rate of 20%. There was also a statistically significant difference in consumption between residents in the urban and rural areas. People in the rural areas had a higher proportion of drinkers (35%) than those in the urban centres (27.4%). This was significant (x^2 = 14.64, $p<0.001$).

BEVERAGE PREFERENCE

Table 2 shows that, among current drinkers, the alcoholic beverage taken most by both males and females respondents was beer (65.0%), followed by palmwine (53.3%), *burukutu* (36.5%), and *ogogoro* (35.1%),

TABLE 2. **Type of alcoholic beverages consumed by male and female current drinkers**

Type of beverage	Gender	n	Yes	Total
Wine	Male	452	25.2	26.6
	Female	205	29.8	
Beer	Male	452	71.2	65.0
	Female	205	51.5	
Liquor	Male	447	24.6	23.0
	Female	204	19.6	
Burukutu	Male	432	38.4	36.5
	Female	193	32.1	
Palmwine	Male	446	54.5	53.3
	Female	199	50.8	
Ogogoro	Male	445	35.1	35.1
	Female	196	35.2	

Note: Percentages are based on the number of valid responses.

with the least often consumed beverages being wine (29.8%) and liquor (23%). Except for *ogogoro* and wine, male drinkers were slightly more likely to consume the beverages which were consumed by higher percentages of females.

DRINKING PATTERNS BY GENDER AND AGE

Respondents were considered to be frequent drinkers if their drinking occasions occurred more than once a month and infrequent if the occasions were less than once a month. Light drinkers were those who consumed less than 5 drinks in a typical drinking day and heavy drinkers were those who consumed 5+ drinks on such days. Table 3 shows the percentage of those who represent different levels of drinking that may occur within a community by gender, across various age groups.

TABLE 3. **Frequency of drinking by gender and age (%)**

	Male			Female		
	18-29 years (n=221)	30-44 years (n=361)	45+ years (n=338)	18-29 years (n=303)	30-44 years (n=314)	45+ years (n=227)
Life time abstainers	10.4	11.4	11.0	16.2	15.0	14.5
Current abstainers	61.1	39.9	34.3	70.0	58.3	56.8
Infrequent light drinker	1.4	4.7	2.7	3.3	5.1	1.8
Frequent light drinker	14.0	20.8	20.7	5.0	7.0	10.6
Infrequent heavy drinker	2.7	3.6	5.3	1.7	3.2	2.2
Frequent heavy drinking	10.4	19.7	26.0	4.0	11.5	14.1

Note: Percentages are based on the number of valid responses.

The table shows that the highest proportion of lifetime abstainers and current abstainers being in the group of the 18-29 years. The percentage of both lifetime and current abstainers begins to drop as one moves to the higher age groups. The difference in the drop was however only significant for the current abstainers, this was both in the male (x^2 =41.32 $p<.0001$) and female (x^2 =12.59 $p<.01$) groups. Results for frequent heavy drinking showed that the highest percentage was in the 45+ age group. This difference was also statistically significant in the male and female groups (x^2 =20.57 $p<.0001$ and x^2 =17.84 $p<.0001$, respectively).

GENDER AND SITUATIONAL CONTEXTS OF DRINKING

The frequency of alcohol consumption in different situational contexts by gender is shown in Table 4. Among both male and female drinkers, the

TABLE 4. Gender and frequency of drinking in different contexts among current drinkers (%)

Contexts	Gender	n	Never	< Monthly	Monthly	Weekly	Daily or nearly daily
During meals	Male	445	64.7	11.0	8.5	10.8	4.9
	Female	197	64.0	18.8	6.1	7.1	4.1
At party	Male	445	18.9	48.5	20.9	8.5	3.1
	Female	203	17.7	59.6	12.8	7.9	2.0
In own home	Male	455	42.4	18.5	10.1	15.8	13.2
	Female	201	36.8	23.4	11.9	15.9	11.9
At friend's house	Male	449	35.4	32.7	15.6	11.4	4.9
	Female	200	35.0	41.5	14.0	7.0	2.5
At workplace	Male	438	79.0	8.9	3.4	3.7	5.0
	Female	194	84.5	5.2	2.1	1.5	6.7
At bar	Male	445	42.7	19.8	8.8	11.2	17.5
	Female	196	62.8	12.8	4.6	5.1	14.8
At restaurant	Male	445	63.4	21.1	6.3	5.2	4.0
	Female	197	77.7	14.7	4.1	1.0	2.5

highest percent indicated drinking at a party, followed by drinking in a friend's house, own home and at a bar. The context in which daily or near-daily drinking occurred most was at a bar followed by drinking in own home. At a glance the table shows that the percentages of males and females that indicated drinking during meals, at a party and at a friend's house were quite similar. Greater differences between males and females were seen in the context of drinking in own home, bar, and restaurant. It was, however, only in the context of own home, that there was a higher percentage of women. The weekly and daily frequencies of drinking by females, however, were not significantly different from those of males.

Binomial logistic regression analyses were performed using the likelihood to drink in different contexts as the outcome variable. There were seven predictors: gender, residence, marital status, educational level, income, religion and age. For the independent factors that had more than two categories, dummy variables were created to allow for the capture of the demographic characteristics that would predict drinking in the different situations. The dummy variables created for inclusion in the analysis included: Age1 and Age2, which differentiated between the three age groups: 18-29 years, 30-44 years, and the reference category aged 45+. For the household income, two dummy variables were created: Income1 and Income2 to designate the high and middle income groups; the reference category for these variables was the low income group. For education we had Educ1 and Educ2 for no education and less than 9 years of education, with the group with 10 years or more as reference category. As the number of respondents in the different categories of marital status were small in some of the cells, marital status was collapsed to a dichotomy: married or cohabiting were placed in the category of married, and the others into "not married." The "not married" group was used as the reference category. Religious preference was also collapsed into two categories of "Christian" and "Others". The reference category for religious preference was "Others".. All the variables were entered as categorical variables.

The result of the regression analyses for the different situational contexts are shown in Table 5. Drinking context was the outcome measure, and with the inclusion of the dummy variables there were ten predictors, namely: gender, residence, income1, income2, educ1, educ2, age1, age2, religious preference and marital status. Results show that drinking during meals was best predicted by taking into account age and income. The 18-29 and 30-44 age groups were less likely to drink during meals than the 45+ group, and being in the high or middle income categories made it more likely that an individual would report drinking in this context. This model was statistically significant (x^2 =31.81, $p<.001$, with Negelkerke R^2 =0.083), indicating that the predictors as a set reliably distinguished drinking in the context of having meals.

Chi-square analysis revealed significant differences in the frequency of occurrence of drinking during meals on a weekly or more bases. Results showed the low income drinking significantly less frequent than the high and middle income group (x^2 =14.2, $p<.001$). Weekly or more frequency of drinking in this context was not significantly different for the different age groups.

In the context of drinking at a party, the variables included in the model were age1(18-29 years), residence, and educ1 (No education). In predicting drinking at a party, respondents in the 45+ age group were more likely to report drinking than the 18-29 age group. The difference between the 30-44 age group and the 45+ was however not statistically significant. The model correctly predicted drinking in this context 81.4% of the time (x^2 = 20.57, df 1, $p<.05$, with Negelkerke R^2 = 0.053). Chi-square analysis of frequency of drinking weekly or more in this context did not yield any significant difference among the different age groups.

Table 5 shows the regression coefficients, Wald statistics, exponential of B (i.e., the odds ratio), for predictors that were indicative of drinking in each context. Gender was included as a predictor in the context of drinking at home, at the bar, and at a restaurant. Predictors of drinking in one's home included were gender, age and income (x^2 = 27.99, $p<.001$,

TABLE 5.   Logistic regression for drinking in different context

Context	Variable[1]	B	S.E.	Wald	Exp(B)
During meals	Age1: 18-29 years*	-0.562	0.279	4.068	0.570
	Age2: 30-44years**	-0.631	0.205	9.462	0.532
	Income1: High**	0.840	0.344	5.946	2.316
	Income2: Middle***	0.860	0.233	13.615	2.364
At party	Age1: 18-29 years **	-1.068	0.325	10.775	0.344
	Residence: Urban*	-0.523	0.226	5.345	0.593
	Educ1: None*	-0.937	0.416	5.085	0.392
	Income2: Middle**	0.632	0.249	6.466	1.882
At home	Age1: 18-29 years **	-0.773	0.267	8.401	0.462
	Age2: 30-44years **	-0.409	0.199	4.213	0.665
	Gender: Male*	-0.464	0.190	5.985	0.629
At friend's house	Income2: Middle*	0.512	0.249	4.229	1.668
	Marital: Married**	-0.554	0.216	6.565	0.575
In bar	Residence: Urban***	-0.591	0.186	10.901	0.554
	Gender: Male***	0.779	0.188	17.161	2.178
At restaurant	Residence: Urban**	0.616	0.197	9.746	1.852
	Income1: High**	0.701	0.354	3.952	2.015
	Marital: Married*	-0.511	0.227	5.083	0.600
	Gender: Male***	0.764	0.224	11.652	2.418
	Educ1: None**	-1.231	0.329	14.153	0.290
	Educ2: 1-9 years**	-1.008	0.281	12.848	0.365

[1]Reference categories are as follows: Gender: Female; Age: 45+ years; Residence: Rural; Education: 10+ years; Income: Low; Marital status: All others
*$p<.05$; **$p<.01$; ***$p<.001$

Negelkerke R^2 = .059). Women were more likely to drink in this context than men. Also the 45+ age group were more likely to report drinking more in this context than those in either the 18-29 or the 30-44 year age group. Likewise those in the middle income bracket were nearly twice as likely to drink in this context than those in the low income group. Analysis of weekly or more frequent drinking in this context revealed a significant difference for age (x^2 = 8.38, $p<.05$) and income (x^2 = 6.20, $p<.05$). The gender difference in frequency of drinking on a weekly or more basis was not statistically significant.

Logistic regression analysis showed that males were twice as likely to report drinking at a bar and restaurant than females. Drinking at a bar was almost twice as likely to be reported by respondents in the rural area as respondents in the urban area, whereas drinking in a restaurant was nearly twice as likely to occur in the urban as in the rural area. Also predictive of drinking in the restaurant was marital status: married people were nearly 40% less likely to drink in a restaurant than unmarried people.

DISCUSSION

The basic thrust of this work was to describe alcohol consumption patterns in general and its occurrence in different situational contexts more specifically. Of interest was how the situational context is related to certain demographic characteristics of the drinker. Here we have adopted a descriptive population perspective of drinking location. Differences in the patterns and intensity of alcohol consumption in Nigeria are determined by such factors as gender, age, income, marital status and area of residence, as selected demographic variables in the survey have shown. Although parties, friend's house and bars were venues that experienced the highest percentage of people indicating that they drink, variations between the contexts depends to a large extent on the demographic characteristics of individuals that patronize these venues.

The results of the study found a significant gender difference in the number of current drinkers, with males having a higher proportion. These results suggest that drinking is primarily a male behaviour. But more importantly, women's consumption patterns are different from men's. The gender dimension of alcohol consumption in Nigeria cannot be divorced from the socio-cultural setting in Nigeria where drinking by women is generally not approved. It is within this framework that the gender issues in alcohol consumption in Nigeria can be understood. For example, whereas the negative and often destructive effects of alcohol abuse generally are increasingly a topical concern in Nigeria, the view that alcohol abuse has different consequences for different gender and social categories is still not very clear to many, including policy makers and scholars. Nevertheless, in view of their roles in production and distribution of alcohol beverages, especially the traditional alcohol beverages, women are not as distanced from alcohol use as may be interpreted from the results of the survey. The pattern presented in Table 3 does point to the fact that women exhibit a similar pattern of drinking across the different age groups. This table shows the percentages of women heavy drinking doubling as one moves from the 18-29 to the 30-44 year age group, and further increasing with the 45+ age group. This table further points out that when drinking does occur, the tendency is for it to be frequent, (irrespective of the individual's gender). Additionally nearly half of the people that do drink are likely to engage in frequent heavy drinking.

Binomial regression analyses revealed gender as a predictive factor in the context of drinking at home, bar and restaurant. As one would have expected, women tended to drink more at home than the men. This may be more as a result of the fact that women, by reason of their role as caretakers of the home and children, tend to spend more time at home; thus the drinking, if it occurs, would be in this context. However, the frequency of females drinking weekly or more in this context did not differ significantly from that of males.

The bar is still considered a male venue and women who go there alone are few and largely outnumbered by males. More often than not the women who drink at the bar do so in the company of men. This, then, may explain the higher ratio of males to females who drink in this context. It should, however, be pointed out that the women that do drink in these venues do not differ significantly in frequency of drinking from their male counterparts. By implication, more men drink at the bar, but the few women that do visit the bars to drink visit these locations just as frequently as their male counterparts.

Likewise, drinking in a restaurant is to a considerable degree a reflection of the individuals that visit these places. In the Nigerian context restaurants are seen, more or less, as a place visited by males who are not currently in a resident marital relationship. Not being in such a relationship, they would tend to eat out more and this often would be in a restaurant, in the process also requesting alcoholic drinks. It is worth noting here that gender was not seen as predictive of alcohol consumption during meals. It is only predictive in the context of restaurants, probably because women who drink during meals probably do so more often in the confines of their own home, either together with their partners or alone. Though more and more women are getting into career jobs, many still prefer to eat food they cooked and therefore are less likely to visit restaurants to eat out as often as their male counterparts. When they do eat out it would often be during office hours. As drinking during work is not considered appropriate and again that the social sanctions for so doing are more grievous for females this may act as further deterrent to their drinking, at this time or context. Notable also is that in terms of beverage preference, wine is the preferred by women more. Wine is not served in many restaurants, and when it is, often it is not served/ordered in glasses. This poses certain inconveniences if one was to then order wine with meals, particularly with a meal taken during office lunch break. Ordering a bottle of wine to go with one's meal would necessitate having to either finish the bottle there, which may not have been the intention, or having to take it back to the office or leave the remainder at the restaurant. Carrying it to the office would carry the risk of being socially branded, whereas leaving it behind would be considered an economic waste.

Christianity and Islam are the two most dominant religions, and there are many that claim to be deeply committed to them. These religions have greatly influenced different aspects of the people's lives, as evident in the occurrence of religiously oriented conflicts and crises. They have also influenced people's drinking behaviour. Both are intolerant of consumption of alcohol, but Islam more so than Christianity. This is not the same for the individuals who practice other forms of religion where rituals involved often include use of alcoholic beverages as an offering, used in appeasing the gods. On the other hand, most members of Christian denominations and Islam would not want to be publicly identified with the use of alcohol. The Christian denominations in Nigeria include many which favour abstinence. In parts of Nigeria the dominance of Muslims has meant that alcohol is formally forbidden. The institution of *Sharia* law in certain states in the country, particularly in the ones bordering the Middle Belt region, has resulted in punitive measures being put in place to control the production, sale and consumption of alcoholic beverages. By implication, the laws make one more conscious of one's consumption, and in that case a drinker either consciously cuts down on his drinking or does not accurately report the consumption. The rates of alcohol consumption thus recorded from the Middle Belt or North Central zone may actually have been affected by this. It is possible that the rates obtained in this zone in general, and among Muslims more specifically, are underestimated.

The influences of social support such as familial and community relationships also affects alcohol consumption. The survey shows that those who were cohabiting, single or married have lower rates for alcohol consumption than those who were widowed. The highest proportions of alcohol consumption were found in the divorced and separated. Cross tabulations carried out showed that more than 80 percent of the separated respondents consumed 5 or more drinks on a typical drinking day. It raises the question of the role that drinking may have played in the separation or divorce. Since the study is cross-sectional, however, it cannot be determined whether it is the drinking that led to the separation and divorce, or the separation and divorce that led to the drinking. The small number of respondents in each of these categories also imposes additional limitations on the inferences that can be drawn in this regard.

The survey shows that the percentage of individuals that drink increases with age. It would appear that as individuals move away from parental control they move closer to and interact more frequently with peer groups, which is a risk factor for increased alcohol consumption. Or it could be that they are now more independent socially and financially, and therefore can afford to do so. It may also be a continuation of the traditional patterns of drinking, whereby drinking was seen as something that elders or people high in the social hierarchy of the society had access to and control over. The respondent's age was predictive of drinking in the contexts of drinking at home, at a party and during meals. In each of these situations the older age group had greater odds of drinking. Doing so weekly or more often was found significant only in the context of drinking in one's home.

Results from this study call for revisiting the thesis of heavier drinking occurring in the urban centers, possibly as a result of the decline in the influence of the extended family and community and the increase salience of peer groups. This effect of urbanization found in earlier studies may refer to drinking among youth, where peer influence seems greatest, and monitoring by parents and other people is a bit relaxed. Different factors may however be at play in the older population, causing the drinking patterns observed in this work. It is possible that economic change has loosened and reorganized the social networks surrounding drinking in the village so that the independence and anonymity experienced in the urban areas is desired and pursued by those in the rural area. With less personal economic activities occurring in the rural area, the tendency is for people to have more time to initiate activities and engage in programmes that may involve social gatherings. These gatherings may be in groups that serve alcohol, particularly as it is regarded as a social lubricant necessary to enhance the social environment in each of the groups. It is possible that the drinking in the rural area is as a result of greater opportunity for people to meet more often in a relaxed atmosphere, than is possible in the urban areas. It may be that the traditional communities that sanctioned drinking in certain situations and circumstances have not changed in the concept of drinking in those circumstances, but rather the frequency in which those circumstances occur has increased.

More members of the middle income group in Nigeria indicated drinking more than those in the low income group. Income was seen as predictive of frequency of drinking during meals, in one's own home, at a friend's house, and at a restaurant. During meals, drinking was more likely in the middle and the high income groups than the lower income group. When considering frequency of drinking in this context however the lower income bracket did so at a significantly less "weekly or more" frequency. A similar pattern was observed for drinking in the context of one's home. Thus, the higher income was predictive of drinking in this context.

The majority of male and female current drinkers in Nigeria drank brands of lager beer. This is possibly because of their widespread availability. This may be largely connected to the production and distribution chains; various brands of lager beer are available all over Nigeria, including the rural locations. Comparatively only very few people could afford the luxury of table wine, which in Nigeria is a 'status symbol'. Female drinkers were more likely than males to drink table wine, which is considered less intoxicating. That the figure for females was not higher may reflect lack of access to resources to purchase table wine.

CONCLUSION

This study set out to look at alcohol consumption patterns in Nigeria, with a specific focus on how situational contexts of alcohol consumption relate to certain demographic variables. The cross-sectional nature of the study imposes certain limitations on the inferences of causality that can be drawn. It may be argued that predictions of context of drinking from demographic groups (e.g., by gender, religion or age) may relate more to seeking locations that promote greater alcohol intake. Or it could be that demographic group membership affects the frequency with which one will desire to visit or avoid visiting locations where drinking occurs. The social atmosphere at these various drinking places also deserves some attention, as it may also contribute to the person's consumption: certain environments may actually be more permissive of impulsive behaviours than others, thus affecting the drinking pattern in that context. To clarify the issues of causality, a longitudinal design would be needed. Despite this limitation, however, the cross-sectional design showed that frequency of consumption varies with the drinking context, implying that people are to some degree affected by their drinking environment.

Thus contextualizing the individual's usual consumption in various locations may provide valuable information for evolving better strategies for targeted preventive actions.

Cultural norms and beliefs with regards to drinking in certain locations affect alcohol consumption patterns. It is important that future work examine the effect of cultural variables and the diversity of alcohol consumption patterns and contexts. For a country like Nigeria, with its diverse cultures, research of this nature is crucial in developing effective prevention strategies.

This study focused on the contexts of alcohol consumption and did not assess other dimensions that may influence drinking. For instance, it did not assess the composition of the drinking group or the drinking companions, and the subtle pressures exerted by such groups. These factors have been seen in other studies (Greenfield & Room, 1997; Demers et al., 2003) to relate to the individual's drinking level. More in-depth research will be required to provide a better explanation of drinking among adults in Nigeria.

ACKNOWLEDGEMENTS

The authors would like to thank Isidore S. Obot, Robin Room, Richard Wilsnack and other members of the North Dakota team, and the whole GENACIS membership that saw to the completion of this project. Their comments, suggestions and support were of immense help. We are greatly indebted to the Federal Office of Statistics, Nigeria for releasing their enumerators to assist in data collection.

REFERENCES

Ahmed, M.H. (1986). Drug abuse as seen in the University Department of Psychiatry, Kaduna, Nigeria in 1980–1984. *Acta Psychiatric Scandinavica,* **14**(1), 98–101.

Ahmed, M.H.(1989). Drug abuse, women and society, some socio-demographic characteristics of female cases in the University department of Psychiatry, Kaduna, Nigeria in 1980-1986. *West African Journal of Medicine* **8**(4), 241–245.

Akerele, A.O. (1993). Supply of alcohol: a major determinant of alcohol consumption and abuse. In I.S. Obot (ed.), *Epidemiology and Control of Substance Abuse in Nigeria* (pp. 45–51). Jos: Centre for Research and Information on Substance Abuse.

Anumoye, A. (1980). Drug use among young people in Lagos. *Bulletin on Narcotics,* **32**(4), 49–45.

Bennet, L.A., Campillo, C., Chandrashekar, C.R. Gureje, O. & Franz P. (1998). Alcoholic beverage consumption in India, Mexico and Nigeria: a cross-cultural comparison. *Alcohol, Health and Research World,* **22**(4), 243–252.

Demers, A., Kairouz, S., Abdul, E.M., Gliksman, L., Newton-Taylor, B. & Marchand, A. (2002). Multi-level analysis of situational drinking among Canadian undergraduates. *Social Science and Medicine,* **55**(3), 417–426.

Ebie, J.C. & Pela, O.A. (1981). Some socio-cultural aspects of the problem of drug abuse in Nigeria. *Drug and Alcohol Dependence,* **8**, 302–306.

Enekwechi, E.E. (1996). Gender differences in motivation for alcohol use among Nigerian university students. *Journal of Alcohol and Drug Education,* **41**(2) 1-10.

Federal Office of Statistics (1985). Industrial Profile 1985. Lagos: FOS.

Federal Office of Statistics (1999). Annual abstract of Statistics. Lagos: FOS.

Gire, J.T. & Dimah, A. (2001). Cultural transformation and the changing pattern of alcohol consumption among the Tiv of Central Nigeria. *African Journal of Drug and Alcohol Studies* **1**(2), 125–137.

Greenfield, T.K., & Room, R. (1997). Situational norms drinking and drunkenness trends in the US adult population 1978-1990. *Addiction,* **92**, **1**, 33-47.

Gureje, O. et al. (1996). Comparison of alcohol and other drugs: experience from the WHO collaborative cross cultural applicability research (CAR) study. *Addiction,* **91**, 1529-1538.

Gureje, O. (1999). Country profile on alcohol in Nigeria. In L. Riley and M. Marshall (ed.), *Alcohol and Public Health in 8 Developing Countries.* (pp. 95–114). Geneva: World Health Organization.

Ibanga, A.K.J. (1997). Epidemiologic trends in drug consumption in Nigeria. Proceedings of the National Workshop on Drug Demand Reduction Policy in Nigerian (pp 61-68). Kuru, Nigeria: National Institute of Policy and Strategic Studies.

Ibanga A.K.J. (1998). Youth, drugs and secret cults. *Journal of the African Council on Narcotics,* **9**, 10-12.

Ibanga, A.K.J. (2002) *Alcohol use: a comparative look at experiences of heavy, moderate and light drinkers.* A paper presented at the sixth Bi-annual conference of the Centre For Research and Information Substance Abuse held in Abuja, Nigeria.

Idowu, A.I. (1987). Prevalence of smoking and drug use among students in Illorin metropolis: implications for counseling. *Illorin Journal of Education,* **3**, 85–92.

Ifabumuyi, O. (1982). Alcoholism: a missed diagnosis. In O. A. Eronosho and N.W. Bell (eds.) *Mental Health in Africa* (pp 115–121). Ibadan: Ibadan University Press

Ikwuagu, P.U., Niftier, J.C. & Isichie, H.V. (1993). Pattern of substances abuse in the psychiatric unit of Jos University Teaching Hospital: a perspective. In: I.S. Obot (ed.), *Epidemiology and Control of Substance Abuse in Nigeria* (pp. 88–94). Jos: Centre for Research and Information on Substance Abuse.

Ikwuesan, B.H. (1994). Drinking problems and the position of women in Nigeria. *Addiction,* **89**, 941-944.

International Council on Alcohol and Addictions. (1988). *Report of a Research Project on Substance Abuse of Some Urban and Rural Areas of Nigeria.* Lausanne: ICAA.

Isichie, H.U., Ikwuagu, P.U., & Eguta, J.O. (1993). Pattern of Alcoholism in Jos, Nigeria and Gastrop-Rausel, West Germany; a comparative study. In I.S.Obot (ed.), *Epidemiology and Control of Substance Abuse in Nigeria* (pp. 123–127). Jos: Centre for Research and Information on Substance Abuse.

Makanjuola. J.D. (1984) The management of alcohol-related problems in general practice in Nigeria. In WHO Management of Alcohol-Related Problems in General Practice. Geneva: WHO.

Maula, J., Lindblad, M., & Tigerstedt, C., eds. (1990). *Alcohol in Developing Countries.* Helsinki: *Nordic Council for Alcohol and Drug Research.* (NAD Publication No. 18).

Ndon, R.J., & Adelekan, M.L. (1996) Psychosocial correlates of substance use among undergraduates in Ilorin University, Nigeria. *East African Medical Journal,* **73**(8), 541-547

Nevadomsky, J. (1982). Self-reported drug use among secondary school students in two rapidly developing Nigerian towns. *Bulletin on Narcotics,* **34**, 12–32.

Netting, R.N. (1964). Beer as a locus of value among the West African Kofyar. *American Anthropologist,* **66**, 826–838.

Lambo, T.A. (1965). Medical and social problems of drug addiction in West Africa. *The West African Medical Journal,* **14**, 236–254.

Obembe, A. (1988). Alcoholism: a ten year hospital survey. *Nigerian Medical Practitioner,* **16**, 181–182.

Obot, I.S. (1993a). Drinking behaviour and attitudes in Nigeria: a general population survey CDS. Monograph series no. 1/93. Jos: University of Jos

Obot, I.S. (1993b). Epidemiology of tobacco and alcohol use in Nigeria. In I.S. Obot (ed.), *Epidemiology and Control of Substance Abuse in Nigeria* (pp 67–87). Jos: Centre for Research and Information on Substance Abuse.

Obot, I.S., Ibanga, A.J. & Karick, H. (2002*). Images of power and success: alcohol promotion and marketing in Nigeria.* Paper presented at Kettil Bruun Society Confercne, Paris 3 – 7th June.

Obot, I.S., Ibanga, A.J., Ojiji, O.O. & Wai, P. (2001). Drug and alcohol consumption by out of school Nigerian adolescents. *African Journal of Drug and Alcohol Studies,* **1**(2), 98 – 109

Obot, I.S. & Olaniyi, A. A. (1991). Drug-related psychotic disorders in four Nigerian hospitals (1984 – 1988). *Nigerian Journal of Psychology,* **8**(1), 13-16.

Odejide, A.O. & Olatawura, M. O. (1997). Alcohol use in Nigerian rural community. *African Journal of Psychiatry,* **1**, 69–74.

Odejide, A.O. (1978). Alcoholism a major health hazard in Nigeria. *Nigerian Medical Journal,* **8**, 230-233.

Ohaeri, J.V. & Odejide, A. O. (1993). Admission for drug and alcohol-related problems in Nigeria psychiatric health care facilities in one year. *Drug and Alcohol Dependence,* **31**, 101–109

Olademeji, B.Y. & Fabiyi, A.K. (1993). Trends in alcohol consumption among Nigerian undergraduates. In I.S. Obots (ed) *Epidemiology and Control of Substance Abuse in Nigeria* (pp. 88–94). Jos: Centre for Research and Information on Substance Abuse.

Oshodin, O.G.(1981). Alcohol abuse: a case study of secondary school students in a rural area of Benin District, Nigeria. *Drug & Alcohol Dependence,* **8**, 207–213.

Oshodin, O.G. (1995). Nigeria. In D.B. Heath (ed.), *International Handbook on Alcohol and Culture* (pp. 213-223). Westport CT: Greenwood Press

Umunna, I. (1967). The drinking culture of a Nigerian community: Onitsha. *Quarterly Journal of Studies on Alcohol,* **28**, 529-537.

Uzor, M. (1999). Nigerian Breweries tops exchange capitalization. *Financial Standard,* 17 December, p. 39.

CHAPTER 8

GENDER, ALCOHOL AND CULTURE IN SRI LANKA

SIRI HETTIGE & DHARMADASA PARANAGAMA

INTRODUCTION AND BACKGROUND

Sri Lanka is a country with a written history of over 2500 years. From the sixth century BC up to the sixteenth century AD, India had a great influence on the cultural outlook of the Sri Lankan population, because of Sri Lanka's proximity to India. Since the 16th century, with the advent of the Western colonial powers, first the Portuguese, then the Dutch and the British, Sri Lanka was exposed to western cultural influence (Ray, 1959; Sarkar, 1957). While pre-colonial cultural patterns, in particular religious traditions, continue to be highly influential, later cultural influences have also become significant in shaping the attitudes, habits and behaviour patterns of many people, particularly in urban areas.

Buddhism, Hinduism and Islam discourage alcohol consumption, while the Roman Catholic and other traditions of Christianity had no such influence. However, toddy produced by tapping flowers of coconut, Palmyra and 'kitul' trees, was popular in all parts of the country, since very early days. Villagers produced it for their own consumption and it was mainly for adult males and not for females and children. Toddy, a fermented beverage with a low alcohol content, was referred to in ancient chronicles and was popular among warriors. Along with toddy, vinegar, jaggery (raw sugar) and trickle (liquid sugar) were produced for household consumption but not on a commercial basis. Today these are produced on a commercial basis by tapping mainly coconut and palmyra trees. Toddy became a commercial product when the British Colonial government introduced taxes on tapped coconut trees and introduced taverns from which the government levied excise duties.

The Portuguese, who colonized coastal areas of Sri Lanka in 1505, had introduced wine drinking. Since then, western powers that ruled the country introduced various types of alcoholic drinks and excise duties, bringing revenue to the state. Popularization of production and drinking of alcoholic beverages increased state revenue and continues to be the case to date.

After independence, the government regularized the production of licit liquor by introducing the Excise Ordinance No. 8 of 1964 (and its amendments). A separate department has also been set up to implement the Excise Ordinance, regularizing production, distribution and sales and collecting government revenue excise duties. A five-fold increase in the government revenue from all excise duties (liquor, tobacco etc.) has been recorded for the ten-year period of 1992-2002, while there was around a three-fold increase in revenue from liquor. Revenue from excise tax has increased from 10.4 billion rupees to 52.3 billion rupees from 1992 to 2002. Similarly revenue from liquor taxes has increased from 3.4 rupees to 10.3 billion rupees during the same period. Excise duties contribute more than 3% to the GDP annually. In other words, excise revenue accounts for more than 1/5th of the total tax revenue of the government. The increase in revenue over the last 10 years was due to increases in consumption and price hikes. The total production of alcoholic beverages in the country during this period had almost doubled (Central Bank, 2002).

There has thus been a rapid increase in alcohol production and consumption over the last ten years. Beer production has increased over fivefold between 1992 and 2002, whereas hard liquor production has increased from 53.4 million liters to 59.6 million liters. Per capita consumption of beer has increased from 0.7 liters to 3.4 liters in the same period. Consumption of hard liquor has also increased steadily during the period. Figures do not include illicit alcohol, which is estimated to be around 50% of total alcohol availability in the country.

Availability of alcoholic drinks for the population is not limited to local licit production. Imports and smuggling of foreign liquor and illicit local brews also come to the market in significant quantities. The police and excise officers arrest people almost every day who are smuggling foreign liquor and distilling and transporting illicit brews in large quantities. Yet it is a thriving and lucrative business, at times supported by corrupt law enforcement officers and local politicians. In the suburbs around Colombo, illicit liquor is produced in large quantities and transported to other urban areas, while in the rural areas it is produced in small quantities, mainly for poor village drinkers.

A policy of popularizing lower-strength liquor like beer was implemented in 1994 by reducing the price of beer to divert hard liquor drinkers to beer. however, it could not achieve the desired objective, as drinkers who are used to hard liquor could not be persuaded to drink beer. If a drinker could not afford licit hard liquor, he would turn to local illicit brews, like 'kasippu', in which alcohol content is very high compared to arrack, the popular licit distilled beverage.

In 2002, Sri Lankan drinkers consumed 56.7 million liters of malt liquor, 56.6 million liters of arrack and 7 million liters of toddy in addition to around 3 million liters of other foreign liquor. However, the quantity of smuggled and illicit liquor in circulation in urban, rural and estate areas might be equal to the quantity of arrack consumed in a given year. Thus the per capita alcohol consumption compiled using licit alcoholic production does not give the true picture in the country, as the per capita consumption may be doubled if illicit liquor is also taken into account.

Apart from local production, both licit and illicit, the supply of liquor for local consumption has been increased by smuggling and imports of liquor. In 2002, around 15.8 million liters of liquor to the value of SLRs. 1,785 million (US $17 million) was imported. This included one million liters of beer, in addition to spirits.

POLICY ON PRODUCTION, SALE, TRANSPORT AND ADVERTISING

The government of Sri Lanka made an attempt in the 1990s to introduce a comprehensive national policy on alcohol for Sri Lanka. This did not, however, result in the formulation and adoption of a national policy, apparently due to the pressure emanating from the liquor industry. So the only legal provision available for controlling liquor production, transport and sales is the Excise Ordinance No. 8 of 1964, the aim of which is to collect taxes on alcohol and tobacco. Earlier, liquor production was a monopoly of the government. However, in the mid-1990s the private sector was also allowed to establish production units, for which licenses have to be obtained from the government. Licensed breweries are given certain guidelines and periodical test checks are being carried out by the Excise Officers.

A license has to be obtained from the Department of Excise to establish sales points and premises of consumption.

(a) for consumption on the premises, such premises should be situated beyond a half mile/500 meter radius from educational institutions and places of religious worship,

(b) for retail off-sales, the premises should be beyond 100 yards/100 meters from educational institutions and place of religious worship.

The issue of licenses is further controlled by taking into account the need for such outlets and the population ratio in that particular area. However, issuing of licenses for retail outlets has been politicized, and bribery and corruption are highly associated with this industry.

Though formally the Commissioner General of Excise can determine the number of licenses to be issued in an area, taking into consideration the following criteria, political interference has curtailed his power, and the decisions are not always made in keeping with the criteria.

- the population and requirements of the area;

- applicant's bank balance, payment of income and turnover taxes, eligibility and ownership of premises;

- reports of the Officer-in-Charge of the Police Station, the Divisional Secretary, and the Officer-in-Charge of the Excise Station of the area that the applicant is the proper person to hold the license, there is no objection from the public for the issue of license and there will be no threat to the maintenance of law and order; and

- the location, size, furnishing, toilets, kitchen, food etc. of the premises relating to hotels and restaurants.

There were over 1880 licensed outlets in the form of restaurants, hotels, rest houses, wine shops, clubs, canteens, taverns etc. by 1995. However, the number of unlicensed outlets increased tremendously all over the country, especially in congested urban areas, in the guise of Chinese restaurants and sports clubs, in addition to thousands of places where illicit liquor is sold, after the liberalization of it in the mid-1990s. There is no reliable data on these various outlets.

Alcoholic beverages widely consumed in Sri Lanka can be categorized as

a) Low alcohol beverages such as beer and toddy, wine with an alcohol content of less than 10%,

b) Strong liquor or spirits such as arrack, gin, brandy etc. with an alcohol content of 35-40%, and

c) Illicit liquor, commonly known as 'kassippu' with a very high alcohol content — around 50%.

Arrack and beer are produced in equal quantities (about 57 million liters per year), whereas other types are produced in much smaller quantities. Production of toddy, which is a fermented traditional brew, amounted to about 7 million liters in 2002.

As mentioned, earlier production and the distribution of alcohol are regulated by the Department of Excise under the Excise Ordinance No. 8 of 1964. According to the Ordinance:

a) All liquor manufactories should be licensed under the Excise Ordinance.

b) Transport of liquor should be done under a licence obtained from the Excise Commissioner.

c) Transport of liquor up to 7500 liters is allowed without a license.

d) A licence for the production of liquor is given only after considering the Government Analyst's Report of the samples.

e) No drinking of alcohol is allowed within the premises of the manufactory.

f) Sale of alcoholic products to children is completely prohibited.

As regards labeling of products, the label used by producers must be approved by the Excise Department and it should carry: (a) the name of the manufactory, (b) the brand, (c) the strength and (d) the price of the product.

The Ordinance also sets limits for alcohol content as follows: foreign liquor (spirits): 37.0% to 45.6 % alcohol; arrack: 33.5% to 36.8% alcohol; beer and toddy: 5.0% to 7.5% alcohol.

There are no restrictions on advertising of liquor in print media and other modes of advertising like billboards, except in the case of electronic media, such as television. Even on television it is not legally banned, but TV and radio stations do not usually carry alcohol advertisements.

Driving under the influence of liquor can be prosecuted under the Motor Traffic Ordinance and under the Offences Committed Under the Influence of Liquor Act No. 41 of 1979. The Traffic Police carry out frequent checks on drunk drivers, as liquor is thought to be a major cause of grave road accidents, which are on the rise. We will return to this issue later in the chapter.

DRINKING CUSTOMS AMONG DIFFERENT POPULATION GROUPS

In Sri Lanka drinking is also associated with gender and culture. As a result, drinking habits, frequency and amount of drinking vary among different ethno-religious communities and socio-economic classes in the country. Frequent heavy drinking could be found among Tamil estate workers, whose educational attainments as well as entertainment facilities are quite low. Gender differences with regard to drinking are not as marked among them, and usually cheap illicit local brews are popular among them. Frequent drinking could also be found among Roman Catholic and other Christian populations found to the north of Colombo City. This community is more westernized and largely English-educated and most of them are engaged in government service and business activities. Many females in this community are also exposed to drinking, compared to other parts of the country, as serving liquor in households is a custom among them. Illicit liquor is also popular in these areas.

Drinking is not as heavy and frequent in other parts of the country, where the population is mainly Buddhist. Female drinking is negligible. However, heavy drinking and alcoholism is associated with low education, hard manual work and poverty in these areas. Some urban females drink beer or wine at social events, which upper class females frequently attend.

Drinking among teenagers is not very common, as parental care is high and culturally children are not used to taking drinks in the presence of parents or respected elders, even at a party. The law prohibits selling drinks to teenagers, those below 18 years of age. On the other hand, drinking is spreading among youth, particularly in urban areas. Though drinking is common among office workers, no one is allowed to take drinks during office hours and no one i supposed to come to the office after drinking. Many office workers have drinks with co-workers at bars and restaurants after work.

ALCOHOL RELATED PROBLEMS

Alcohol is one of the main causes of chronic liver disease and cirrhosis of the liver, but data on morbidity and mortality that can be directly related to alcohol consumption are not readily available. Some of the data could be collected from the Department of the Registrar General, the Department of Police, the Department of Health (Health Statistics Unit) and the Department of Prisons. The major problem a researcher faces in this regard is the delays in publishing annual administrative reports of relevant departments, from which we have to collect data. Unpublished data available in public institutions cannot be readily accessed.

As the available data show, the rate (per 100,000 population) of morbidity and mortality caused by liver cirrhosis and other chronic liver diseases associated with alcohol is on the rise. The rate of cases of diseases of the liver per 100,000 population has increased from 38.5 to 125.2 and deaths from liver diseases from 3.8 to 15.2 during the period of 1975 to 2002. The rate of this disease is high in heavy drinking areas such as the Up Country plantation sector and in the Catholic and Christian areas of North of Colombo (Gampaha and Puttalam Districts) (see also Hettige, 1988 and Dept. of Health Services, 2002). It is noteworthy that the reported cases of alcoholic psychosis have also increased in recent years. For instance, the rate of alcoholic psychosis per 100,000 population has increased from 36.2 in 1990 to nearly 58 in 1995. This is an increase over 60% over a five year period. Nearly one out four mental disorders in Sri Lanka is due to alcohol (Dept. of Health Services, 2002).

Data on deaths caused by injury and poisoning that can be directly related to alcohol are not readily available. The number of homicides, including deaths from injury purposefully inflicted, and deaths caused by accidental poisoning are high. Deaths caused by alcohol poisoning are included in the accidental poisoning. While homicides increased from 1085 in 1985 to 1351 in 1995, alcoholic poisoning increased from 539 to 652 over the same period. These include cases of alcohol poisoning from contaminants which is a common occurrence among consumers of illegally produced alcohol.

And finally to look at motorcar accidents. Available data shows that traffic accidents have increased steadily in recent years. For instance, the rate of traffic accidents per 100,000 population has increased from 202 in 1990 to 211 in 1993. It is significant that the rate of driving under the influence of alcohol has increased form 8.9 in 1990 to 20.7 in 1993, a more than 100 % increase.

GENACIS SURVEY

The objectives of the GENACIS study in Sri Lanka have been:

i) To compare the patterns of drinking between men and women,

ii) To examine the prevalence of drinking problems among men and women,

iii) To assess the level of drinking among men and women,

iv) To carry out cross-national comparisons of drinking problems and heavy drinking occasions,

v) To contribute to the development of alcohol epidemiology involving comparisons between men and women in different cultural contexts, and

vi) To gauge public opinion on certain policy related issues.

METHOD

The main instrument of data collection was the expanded core questionnaire developed by the international GENACIS research team. The questionnaire was suitably modified, taking into consideration specific local conditions. Having been adapted to suit the local conditions, the questionnaire was translated into Sinhala and Tamil, the two native languages. The local language versions were translated back into English in order to ensure that there are no serious distortions made in the translation process. A few questions on alcohol policy issues were added to the expanded core questionnaire used.

SAMPLE

Seventeen out of 25 districts in the island were selected and stratified into four socio-economic zones, which are also identified as agro-ecological zones. The population of the districts in these zones was again stratified into three sectors, namely urban, rural and estate, and each sector by ethnicity, namely Sinhala, Tamil and Moor. The districts that were not considered in the sample selection process are from the North and East of the country, where the security situation was not favourable for conducting the survey. The population in Zone 1 is predominantly urban, whereas Zones 2 and 3 are predominantly rural. The estate population mainly falls into Zone 4. The latest Census of Population data have been used in the selection of the sample. The most recent census was conducted in 2001.

A representative sample of 1200 respondents was used in this survey. A stratified multistage sampling technique with probability proportion to the size of population (PPS) and cluster sampling techniques have been employed in selecting the 1200 respondents. The primary sampling unit was the household. The respondent from the household was selected randomly from among all the members of the family aged 15 and above.

PROCEDURE

First, at least one district was selected to represent each zone. Secondly, two Divisional Secretariat Divisions (DSD) were selected from each selected district with PPS. Thirdly, two Grama Niladhari Divisions (GND) (village headman division) were selected at random (SRS) from each selected DSD. The required number of households was selected employing a systematic sampling technique. Finally, respondents who were aged 15 years and above were selected at random using the list of household members prepared by the enumerator/interviewer.

RESULTS

In this section we provide the main results of the survey. The areas covered in the analysis were:

a) Demographic characteristics of the respondents,

b) Drinking and abstinence,

c) Frequency and quantity of drinking,

d) Characteristics of drinkers

e) Reasons for abstinence,

f) Religion, ethnicity and drinking,

g) Age at first drink,

h) Social context of drinking and

i) Opinions on policy issues.

DEMOGRAPHIC CHARACTERISTICS OF THE SAMPLE POPULATION

Demographic characteristics of the sample population by gender are given in Table 1. Out of the enumerated respondents, there were 698 (50.6%) males and 593 (49.4%) females, with a sex ratio of 1.02 males for each female, indicating that there was no significant gender bias in the sample. The Census of Population conducted in 2001 (a partial census) indicates a sex ratio of 0.98.

With regard to the age structure, nearly one out of four respondents were in the younger age group of 15-29 years, and three out of five were in the age group of 30-59 years. The older respondents aged 60 and above consisted of around 14%, with more old male persons among respondents. Mean ages of males and females were 42.6 years and 40 years, respectively. Both the ethnic and the religious composition of the GENACIS sample and the Census of Population 2001 are similar, pointing to a high degree of accuracy and representativeness of the sample.

In Sri Lanka there is a high correlation between ethnicity and religion of the population. Almost all the Moors are Muslim or Islamic by religion. The Catholic community consists of converts from the Sinhalese and Tamil ethnic groups, who are mostly Buddhists and Hindus, respectively. Sinhala Buddhists form the majority of the population, while the size of the Tamil-Hindu population and Muslim-Malay Islamic population is almost equal.

TABLE 1. **Number and percent of respondents by demographic characteristics**

Demographic characteristics	Male (n =608)	Female (n =593)
Age	%	%
18-29	24.7	26.0
30-44	33.6	37.3
45+	41.8	36.8
*Mean	44.11	42.68
SD	15.98	15.65
Residence		
Rural	78.1	75.5
Urban	21.9	24.5
Education		
No schooling	2.8	6.7
Less than 10 yrs of schooling	67.4	70.2
More than 10 yrs. of schooling	29.8	23.1
Religion		
Buddhist	80.1	80.4
Hindu	8.4	7.3
Muslim	6.6	7.9
Roman Catholic & other Christian	4.6	4.0
Other	0.3	0.3
Marital status		
Married	71.1	73.7
Living with a partner	0.2	0.5
Widow	3.0	11.6
Divorced	0.0	0.5
Separated	0.3	2.4
Never Married	25.5	11.3

Note: In calculating the age mean, the oldest age group (45+) was taken as 45-79 years, covering 99.3% of the respondents.

As the literacy rate of Sri Lanka is high (92.5 for males and 87.9 for females) the proportion of respondents who had no formal education was very low. Educational attainments vary by ethnicity. The proportion of respondents who had no formal education was higher among Tamils than in other ethnic groups. More than half in all the ethnic groups had up to 10 years of schooling.

Altogether, 72% of the respondents were married, while 18% were never married. Those who lived with a partner without legally marrying were very few (0.3%). Divorced and separated respondents, 0.2% and 1.3% respectively, were also few, though the proportion of widowed respondents (7.2%) seemed to be high. In Sri Lanka living with a partner without getting legally married or marrying several times are not culturally much accepted. At the same time, unlike in the West, in Sri Lanka, overt romantic relations among married couples are not given explicit expression due to cultural norms prevailing among the majority of the people, particularly in rural areas.

A majority of the households consisted of husband and wife and their children. Very often unmarried adult children live with their parents, and parents of the married couple also live in the same household, as it is a social obligation and a responsibility of the children to support their parents. Most adults in Sri Lanka do not enjoy old age pensions, as is usually the case in developed countries. Unemployed youth do not receive any unemployment benefit from the state, forcing them to depend on families for their sustenance. A little less than half of the households (48%) in the sample had an income less than Rs. 5,000 per month (approximately 50 US dollars) and are assumed to be poor. A similar proportion belong to the lower and upper middle class. At the same time it may be said that nearly one out of four households were below the poverty line, as their monthly income was below 3,000 rupees. Only 2.5% of the households belong to the upper class with a monthly income of above Rs. 25,000.

Two out of five (40%) respondents were engaged in household work. Respondents engaged in occupations with a higher income (Administrative, professional and large business) consist of around 2%, and around 11 % were engaged in middle level occupations (small business, technicians, clerical and teaching). Around 30% were in low income-generating occupations, such as labourers, farmers, salesmen etc. The socio-economic and demographic profile of the sample population given above points to the fact the sample selected for the survey represents the general population in the country, except the people living in the North and East. It can thus be assumed that the picture emerging from the present survey corresponds to the conditions prevailing in the country.

DRINKING AND ABSTINENCE

Table 2 gives the drinking status of the respondents. It is clear that 30% of the adults (aged above 15 years) are current users of alcoholic beverages at the time of the survey, indicating that a majority (70%) are current abstainers. The current abstainers include both those who had ever taken a drink, but are currently abstaining, and those who had never taken any alcoholic beverage in their lifetime. It is clear that nearly half of the adults in Sri Lanka had taken any alcoholic beverage, and of these more than one-third had given up drinking at the time of the survey.

TABLE 2. **Number and percent of respondents by drinking status and gender**

Drinking status	Male (n = 608)	Female (n = 593)	Total (n =1201)
Current user	53.1	6.4	30.1
Lifetime abstainers	19.2	86.3	52.4
Ever drinkers, now not drinking	27.6	7.3	17.6

Of the 30% of the respondents who are current drinkers, a large majority (90%) are males. Only 10% of the current drinkers are females. Out of all the male respondents, more than half (53%) are current drinkers. It is also clear that over 80% of the males had taken alcohol in their lifetime, but a third of them (27.6% of the whole sample) had given up drinking. Females in Sri Lanka are not quite so used to drinking, as only 13.7% of the females had ever taken an alcoholic drink. Out of them, only 6.4% are still taking drinks and others (7.3%) had given up drinking. It may be assumed that nearly one out of three in the population (age 15 and above) are current drinkers, while drinking among females is almost negligible. Nearly nine out of ten females are lifetime abstainers.

FREQUENCY AND QUANTITY OF DRINKING

Drinking pattern by demographic characteristics of the respondents is given in Table 3.

On a given day 70% of the respondents said that they had not taken a drink during the last 12 months. By gender, 47% of males and a very large majority of females (93.6%) had not taken a drink during the last 12 months. It means that more than one-half of the males had taken drinks during the reference period, against 7% of the females.

Current drinkers were classified in two ways. Considering the quantity of drinking, current drinkers were classified as *light drinkers and heavy drinkers*. Those who had taken less than 60 grams a day were classified as light drinkers and those who had taken more than 60 grams as heavy drinkers. Again, considering the frequency of drinking, each of the light and heavy drinkers were classified as *frequent drinkers and infrequent drinkers*. Those who drank more than three times a week were regarded as frequent drinkers and those who drank less than three times a week as infrequent drinkers.

Culturally female drinking is not sanctioned in many situations, unless the woman comes from a certain socio-cultural background. As a result, female drinking is very low. Only 6.4% of females were current drinkers, compared to 53% of males. Gender specific drinking patterns are given in Table 4.

TABLE 3. Drinking pattern and demographic characteristics (%)

Demographic characteristics	Male				Females		
	Abstainers	Weekly	Usual quantity (3 + drinks)	Ever 5+ drinks	Abstainers	Weekly	Usual quantity 3 + drinks
	n=117	n=106	n=223	n=101	n=512	n=1	n=6
Age							
18-29	39.3	9.4	21.1	15.8	26.0	0.0	16.7
30-44	23.1	48.1	46.2	54.5	36.3	100.0	50.0
45-+	37.6	42.5	32.7	29.7	37.7	0.0	33.3
Residence							
Rural	71.8	85.8	84.8	86.1	77.7	0.0	66.7
Urban	28.2	14.2	15.2	13.9	22.3	100.0	33.3
Education							
No schooling	0.9	4.7	3.6	5.0	7.0	0.0	16.7
< 10 yrs of schooling	55.6	83.0	74.0	76.2	71.7	100.0	50.0
>/= 10 yrs of schooling	43.6	12.3	22.4	18.8	21.3	0.0	33.3
Religion							
Buddhist	69.2	86.8	84.8	82.2	81.3	100.0	66.7
Hindu	5.1	9.4	10.8	11.9	7.2	0.0	16.7
Muslim	22.2	0.0	0.9	0.0	8.8	0.0	0.0
Roman Catholic & other Christian	3.4	3.8	3.6	5.9	2.7	0.0	16.7
Marital status							
Married	57.3	81.1	74.0	76.2	73.4	0.0	66.7
Living with a partner	0.0	0.0	0.4	0.0	0.6	0.0	16.7
Widow	0.9	2.8	2.2	1.0	11.9	0.0	0.0
Divorced	0.0	0.0	0.0	0.0	0.6	0.0	0.0
Separated	0.0	0.9	0.4	0.0	2.3	0.0	0.0
Never Married	41.9	15.1	22.9	22.8	11.1	100.0	16.7

*Percentages do not add up to 100 because categories overlap

A salient feature in Sri Lankan gender-specific drinking is the absence of heavy or light frequent drinking among female drinkers. There was only one female who said that she was a heavy drinker but infrequent. An overwhelming majority of the female drinkers, 97.4%, were infrequent light drinkers. Most of these females had taken alcohol less than 3-6 times during the last 12 months, and the largest drink at a time was 12 grams or

TABLE 4. Typology of drinkers by gender and type of drinking (current drinkers only, in percent)

Typology of drinking: Frequency and quantity	Male (n = 323)	Female (n = 38)	Total (n = 361)
Infrequent light drinking	62.8	97.4	66.5
Infrequent heavy drinking	22.3	2.6	20.2
Frequent light drinking	3.4	0.0	3.0
Frequent heavy drinking	11.5	0.0	10.2

less. More than half of them had taken just a sip, probably at a function, a wedding or a birthday party, just to keep company.

With regard to males, heavy frequent drinking was observed among 11.5% of male drinkers. A majority of male drinkers, nearly two out of three male drinkers, were light infrequent drinkers. Heavy drinking (frequent or infrequent) was reported only among 1/3rd of male drinkers.

Gender and age: The pattern of alcohol consumption, level and frequency of drinking, by gender and broad age groups is given in Table 5. These data indicate that female drinking in Sri Lanka is a recent phenomenon, confined to a certain group of females, and that alcoholism among Sri Lankan females is not so evident as in the West.

No incidence of heavy drinking, frequent or infrequent, is reported among females in the survey. Almost all the female drinkers (91%) were light infrequent drinkers, and a majority of them came from the younger and middle-aged groups. Frequent drinking was reported only among a middle-aged group of females. As habitual drinking was non-existent among females in Sri Lanka, their drinking was confined to social occasions, such as a wedding ceremony, a birthday party, or a social get together at the work place. Unlike in the West, they were not used to drinking at a pub with a partner or friends.

With regard to males' drinking patterns, although more than half of the males take drinks at various levels and frequencies, only a small proportion

TABLE 5. Level and frequency of drinking by gender and age

| Level of drinking | Male | | | | Female | | | |
	18-29 (n=153)	30-44 (n=205)	45+ (n=253)	Total (n=611)	18-29 (n=153)	30-44 (n=219)	45+ (n=218)	Total (590)
Abstainers	48.4	34.1	55.7	46.6	93.5	92.7	95.9	94.1
Infrequent light	37.9	32.2	24.1	30.3	6.5	5.9	4.1	5.4
Infrequent heavy	11.8	20.5	9.1	13.6	0.0	0.0	0.0	0.0
Frequent light	1.3	4.9	7.9	5.2	0.0	1.4	0.0	0.5
Frequent heavy	0.7	8.3	3.2	4.3	0.0	0.0	0.0	0.0

of them (8%) report heavy frequent drinking. However, nearly 18% were used to frequent drinking, while over 82% used to take alcohol infrequently. Heavy frequent drinking was mainly confined to the middle-aged group of males, whereas light infrequent drinking characterized the younger age cohort. Light frequent drinking was mainly the habit of older age group.

RESIDENCE

The distribution of drinkers by district and gender is important, as drinking patterns vary by regions. In general, nearly one out of three adults is a current drinker. Drinking is quite prevalent mainly in the Gampaha district (50%), as a majority of the Catholic and Christian populations is concentrated in this district and in the plantation district of Nuwara-Eliya (45.7%). It should be noted here that the drinking habit among plantation workers goes back to the British colonial period, when commercial production of alcohol became a major source of revenue for the colonial government.

Considering the female drinkers, the highest proportion (43.3%) was also reported from Gampaha, whereas the second highest proportion of female drinkers (18.8%) was reported from the plantation district of Nuwara-Eliya, in which most of the estate Tamils were concentrated. The highest proportion of male drinkers was also reported from Gampaha and Nuwara-Eliya. Male drinking was high in highly urban districts like Colombo and highly rural districts like Polonnaruwa.

RELIGION AND ETHNICITY

In Sri Lanka drinking varies by ethnicity and religion also. Religion and ethnicity in Sri Lanka is highly correlated, as shown above. Culturally, drinking is not a socially approved custom among Sinhalese, Hindus and Muslims, though it is among Catholic and Christian households in Sri Lanka.

It is clear that drinking among Muslims/Moors is quite low compared to other ethno-religious groups and almost all of these drinkers are 'light infrequent drinkers'. Drinking among Sinhalese/ Buddhists is also lower than among Hindu-Tamils. Drinking is quite high among the Sinhala and Tamil Roman Catholic converts. Among the Christian community, 'heavy frequent' (33%) or 'heavy infrequent drinking' (66.7%) was high compared to the level of heavy frequent drinking among Sinhala/Buddhists (10.5%) and Tamil/Hindus (10.3%). Heavy infrequent drinking was high among Hindus (23.1%) compared to the Buddhists (19.7%). The majority of all these communities were light infrequent drinkers.

Frequent drinking was common only among males in all the religious communities, as none of the females were frequent drinkers. Almost all female drinkers (except one) were light infrequent drinkers.

By occupation heavy-frequent drinking among males was mainly found among farmers (39%), unskilled labourers (28%) and skilled labourers (19%). It means that many more poor manual workers tend to be alcoholics than those in other occupations. Drinking among females (light-infrequent) was mainly confined to household workers (67%), clerical (office) workers (15%) and labourers (12%). More of the night time and shift workers were exposed to drinking than others.

At the same time, drinking among males as well as females was positively associated with income. More than 60% of the males whose household income was higher than Rs. 25,000 took alcohol, while it gradually dropped to below 44% at the lowest income level. Drinking among females dropped from 27% in the high-income group to 2.3% in the low-income group. In other words, drinking is more common among upper class women.

It is clear that manual workers and middle level office workers, as well as those in the higher income groups, are more exposed to drinking than others. According to these data, drinking is not much associated with unemployment, as the unemployed probably could not afford it. In Sri Lanka, the unemployed do not have access to unemployment insurance as in the case in most of the developed countries.

Some think that drinking is associated with loneliness. However, it is not so strong in the case of Sri Lankan drinkers. Nearly 70% of the infrequent drinkers never or seldom felt lonely, though it dropped to 57% with regard to heavy frequent drinkers. It may be assumed that heavy drinking was somewhat associated with loneliness, though it is not so strong, in the case of Sri Lanka.

Low alcohol drinks like beer are popular among female drinkers, while a few, probably at higher income levels, had taken wine and whisky at parties. However, a few females had taken hard liquor like arrack and illicit liquor, probably at lower levels of society. Arrack was the most popular liquor, beer being the second preference, among males. In villages, where licit liquor was not easily available, illicit liquor with high alcohol content was also popular among males.

AGE AT FIRST DRINK

Age at first drink often influences the drinker to be a heavy drinker or not. There was only one female who had her first drink at the age of 1 year. Though a majority of the female drinkers (69%) had their first drink during their prime age of 20-34 years, a considerable proportion of females (18%) had their first drink at the age of 15-19 years, that is, during their school days.

Contrary to the female drinking pattern, a majority of the males (63%) got used to drinking during their teenage and prime youth, 10-24 years. It was revealed that heavy frequent drinkers had started to drink when they were teenagers.

REASONS FOR ABSTENTION

There were 629 respondents (117 males and 512 females) who had never taken alcohol, meaning that nearly one out of two respondents abstained from taking alcohol in Sri Lanka. A majority of them were female, as 94% of the females abstained from taking alcohol, compared to 47% of males. Abstainers were asked their reasons for not drinking alcohol (see Table 6 below). More than economic and health factors, self-consciousness and cultural factors played a major role in keeping them as abstainers. Gender differences are not so significant. Over 80% of the both males and females said that they were not interested in drinking and had seen the bad impact of alcohol. This was mainly due to their cultural background. They were brought up in their families not to drink. Religion also played a major role in keeping them abstainers. Fifty to 70 percent of the respondents abstained because alcohol would generate adverse impacts on their day-to-day activities, health and income, thinking that it was a waste of money.

TABLE 6. **Percentage of abstainers by reason for not drinking**
(percentages from total male & female abstainers)

Reasons for not drinking	Male (n=117)	Female (n=512)	Total (n=629)
I have no interest in drinking	89.7	98.4	96.8
I have seen bad examples of what alcohol can do	85.5	90.6	89.7
Drinking is against my religion	70.1	82.8	80.4
I was brought up not to drink	74.4	82.8	81.2
Drinking is too expensive	31.6	36.7	35.8
Drinking is a waste of money	59.0	64.5	63.4
Drinking is bad for my health	70.1	70.1	70.1
My health is bad, and I can't drink	8.5	8.6	8.6
I can't drink because of medication	6.0	2.0	2.7
I am pregnant/trying to get pregnant	0.0	1.0	0.8
I don't like the taste of alcohol	19.7	35.7	32.8
I don't like the effect of alcohol	57.3	63.1	62.0
I have been hurt by someone else's drinking	6.8	7.8	7.6
Drinking would have a bad effect on my activities	53.8	52.0	52.3
I am afraid of being an alcoholic if I drink	41.9	38.3	39.0
No particular reason for drinking	29.1	33.4	32.6

CHARACTERISTICS OF ABSTAINERS

Characteristics of the ex-drinkers and lifetime abstainers are given in Table 7, below. Out of four abstainers, three were lifetime abstainers and

TABLE 7. Percentage of abstainers by demographic characteristics

Demographic characteristics	Ex-drinkers (n=211)	Lifetime abstainers (n=629)	Total (n=840)
Gender			
Male	79.6	18.6	33.9
Female	20.4	81.4	66.1
Age			
18-29	18.0	28.5	25.8
30-44	28.4	33.9	32.5
45+	53.6	37.7	41.7
Educational attainment			
No formal schooling	3.3	5.9	5.2
Primary (1-5 years of schooling)	22.3	17.0	18.3
Secondary (6-10 years of schooling)	46.9	51.7	50.5
Tertiary (GCE A/L)	19.9	21.0	20.7
Higher	3.3	2.1	2.4
Degree	3.3	1.6	2.0
Professional	0.9	0.8	0.8
Ethnicity			
Sinhala	87.2	80.3	82.0
Tamil	7.6	8.1	8.0
Moors	5.2	11.3	9.8
Other	0.0	0.3	0.2
Religious preference			
Buddhist	82.0	79.0	79.8
Hindu	5.7	6.8	6.5
Muslim	5.2	11.3	9.8
Roman Catholic	3.8	1.6	2.1
Other Christian	2.4	1.3	1.5
Other	0.9	0.0	0.2
Residence			
Rural	76.8	73.0	73.9
Estate	4.3	3.7	3.8
Small town	4.3	5.4	5.1
Medium town	4.7	4.6	4.6
City	6.6	7.3	7.1
Large City	3.3	6.0	5.4
Marital status			
Married	75.4	70.4	71.7
Living with a partner	0.0	0.5	0.4
Widow	8.1	9.9	9.4
Divorced	0.0	0.5	0.4
Separated	1.4	1.9	1.8
Never Married	15.2	16.9	16.4
Occupational status			
Voluntarily unemployed	1.4	2.6	2.3
Homemaker	18.0	62.3	51.1
Parental or pregnancy leave	0.0	0.2	0.1
Not working due to illness	6.6	1.1	2.5
Retired	13.7	1.8	4.8
Student	3.3	3.0	3.1
Involuntarily unemployed	4.3	6.2	5.7
Working for pay	52.6	22.8	30.3

one was an ex-drinker. A majority of females were abstainers and a large proportion of these abstainers, four out of five, were lifetime abstainers, while out of male abstainers, a majority, four out of five, were ex-drinkers. Though lifetime abstinence is not age-specific, a large proportion — more than half — of the ex-drinkers were above age 45 years. In Sri Lanka parents think that they must refrain from drinking as their children grow up. As the parents advanced in age and experience more family responsibility they tended to give up drinking. On the other hand, only a little less than half of the lifetime abstainers as well as ex-drinkers had a secondary educational achievement, which indicates that a majority of the abstainers were not highly educated, as expected.

Ethnicity and religious affiliations show that majority of the abstainers were Sinhalese and Buddhists, and most of them were living in the rural sector. Over 70% of the abstainers were married. With regard to occupational status, out of lifetime abstainers, over 62% of were homemakers and another 23% were working for pay. On the other hand, as a majority of ex-drinkers were males, more than half of them were working for pay and around 14% were retired, dropping the proportion of homemakers to a lower level.

SOCIAL CONTEXT OF DRINKING

Respondents in the present study were asked about the freedom for drinking at a given occasion and cultural recognition of drinking in certain contexts. Culturally, taking alcohol in public is not much appreciated. Female drinking even at a party is not recognized as a custom. However, with the ongoing westernization drinking at a party is becoming a common occurrence, as long as it is not a habit. In Sri Lanka parties are not so common. Most of the parties that a common man has to attend once or twice a month are wedding ceremonies, where liquor is served very often. A wife who is against her husband's drinking very often tolerates the husband enjoying a couple of drinks at a party. However, males as well as females did not approve of getting drunk. Almost all specified 'no drinking' for a parent spending time with small children, for a wife having dinner out with husband, for a women out at a bar with friends, for a couple of co-workers out for lunch, with friends after work before going home and when going to drive a vehicle. Drinking was somewhat tolerated for a man, not for a woman, out at a bar with friends, for a husband having dinner out with his wife and with friends at home.

RESPONDENT'S OPINION ON POLICY ISSUES

Respondents in the present study were asked about their opinion on alcohol advertising and the alcohol industry as a source of government income. An overwhelming majority, nine out of ten respondents, was of the opinion that alcohol advertising should not be allowed at all. They were of the opinion (over 95%) that the government should take policy decisions on reducing alcohol production, sale and drinking. Only one out of five approved of the government promoting alcohol as a source of revenue to the state. A strong majority (93%) of the females, who were concerned about the well being of the family, and 76% of the males pointed out that drinking affects peace in the family. More than half of the respondents, 58%, said that it would affect the family income and also create health problems. More males than females were of the opinion that alcohol increases violence and rate of crimes in the country.

CONCLUSION

Commercial production of alcohol in Sri Lanka goes back to the colonial period, commencing in the early 16th century. However, after independence in 1948, the alcohol economy was controlled by the state, which controlled production and sale through a state monopoly. This situation changed in the early 1990's when the state monopoly was privatized. Since then production and sale became highly commercialized, leading to increased production and consumption.

In 1995, beer was promoted by reducing the price and making it available at almost all restaurants, supermarkets, sport meets and clubs, with the intention of reducing the use of hard liquor. However, this objective could not be achieved, as hard liquor consumers did not turn to beer. Instead, more and more new customers were added with the liberalization policy. In Sri Lanka, recent trends indicate that alcohol consumption has a positive association with the rate of crimes, violence, road accidents, alcohol related morbidity and intra-family violence, including child abuse.

At the same time alcohol consumption and abstinence in Sri Lanka are highly related to cultural background, the type of work engaged in, and the gender and social status of an individual. More frequent drinking was reported among the Christian community than among Hindus, Buddhists and Muslims. Although drinking among Muslims was reported to be low, it seems to be under-reported, as they were not ready to concede in public that they take alcohol. Drinking was high among Tamils in the estates and among Sinhalese in urban and highly rural districts. In all the sectors, except among estate Tamil and Christian communities, drinking among females was almost negligible, due to cultural reasons.

On the other hand, Sri Lanka is undergoing rapid change in all spheres of life, largely owing to the open economic policy introduced in 1977. Most of the females, who were confined to household work, cottage industries and village farms prior to 1970s, are now eager to migrate to urban areas and adapt to factory life or migrate to the Middle East as domestic servants, relinquishing family life. Consequently, cultural barriers are breaking down. This process is accelerated by the electronic media that have penetrated even the remote parts of the country.

In the sample there was no gender bias, as both males and females were equally represented. The mean ages of the males and females were 42.6 and 40 years, respectively. The literacy rate of the plantation workers, mainly Tamil, was generally low compared that of others. Marital disruptions in the sample were quite low as in the general population, though widowhood was somewhat high. A majority of the respondents were engaged in household work and low income generating occupations. In general the sample represents a cross section of the total population of the country.

Culturally, drinking in Sri Lanka is mainly confined to males and as a result drinking among females in the sample is almost negligible. While more than half of the males were current drinkers, only 6% of the females were reported as current drinkers. None of the females were heavy drinkers or frequent drinkers. Nearly one out of three males in the country is a current drinker. More than half of the respondents were lifetime abstainers, with wide variation by gender. One out of five males, compared to four out of five females, was an abstainer. Heavy frequent drinking was not widespread in Sri Lanka, as around one out of ten males was found in this category. The majority were light infrequent drinkers.

Drinking in Sri Lanka is gender, ethno-religious and sector specific. Frequent drinking could be found in the plantation and urban sectors, whereas drinking among Moors/Muslims was very low. At the same time drinking was mainly confined to adults, as liquor sale to children is strictly prohibited. Illicit liquor was popular in the low income groups. The majority of the drinkers had their first drink at the age of 20-34 years, and it was found that those who got used to drinking at very early age of life continued to be heavy drinkers. The abstainers had given many reasons for not drinking. With regard to opinion on policy issues a very large proportion of the respondents were against promoting liquor through various types of advertising. Most respondents did not favour the state using alcohol as a major source of revenue.

In conclusion, it is important to note that this study had its share of limitations. For instance, though 1200 households were selected, the sample size was not large enough to fully cover pockets of the population which are exposed to much greater drinking than in the general population. Also, questionnaire surveys like this one cannot collect in-depth data, as the interviewer has limited time to probe into complex issues. It was revealed that some respondents who had been drinking at the time of the interview denied that they take alcohol, due to cultural constraints. (Drinking is not accepted in certain socio-cultural contexts). Some respondents were reluctant to answer a few of the culturally sensitive questions regarding personal life.

ACKNOWLEDGMENTS

We acknowledge the support and advice received from numerous individuals and organizations in conducting the research on which the present chapter is based. The constant encouragement and support we received from Isidore Obot went a long way in facilitating our work. We are extremely grateful to Robin Room for his insightful comments and valuable suggestions on an earlier version of the present chapter. We also note our appreciation of the guidance we received from Sharon Wilsnack, Richard Wilsnack and Arlinda Kristjanson of the University of North Dakota GENACIS research team . Our thanks also go to our research assistants, who did a wonderful job in collecting the necessary household data from different parts of the country.

REFERENCES

ADIC (1994). *Survey on impact of alcohol use on family well being: a study of urban shanty dwellers, Colombo District*. Colombo, Sri Lanka: Alcohol and Drug Information Center.

ADIC (1995a). *Survey of substance use among a selected sample of household in an estate community*. Colombo, Sri Lanka: Alcohol and Drug Information Center.

ADIC (1995b). *Community Survey on Substance Abuse in Seven Districts, Sri Lanka*. Colombo: Alcohol and Drug Information Center.

ADIC (1995c). *Substance use among school children in six districts*. Colombo, Sri Lanka: Alcohol and Drug Information Center.

ADIC (1996). *Opinion of youth regarding alcohol and tobacco advertising*. Colombo, Sri Lanka: Alcohol and Drug Information Center.

Central Bank of Ceylon (2002). *Annual Report*. Colombo: Central Bank of Sri Lanka.

Dept. of Excise (1989, 1990, 1991, 1992, 1993, 1994, 1995). *Annual Reports*. Colombo, Sri Lanka: Department of Excise.

Grant, Marcus (1989). Foreword. In T. Kortteinen (ed.), *State monopolies and alcohol prevention*. Helsinki: The Social Research Institute of Alcohol Studies, Report 181.

Gunasekara, Olcott and M.R.C. Perera (1997). *Survey on assessing the impact of drug use on programmes for alleviating poverty*. Colombo: Sober.

Gunasekara, Olcott (1997). *Alcohol and tobacco in Sri Lanka*. Colombo: Sober.

Hettige, S. T. (1988). Alcohol related problems in Sri Lanka. In A. Erickson (ed), *Alcohol and Drugs*. Colombo: Alcohol and Drug Information Center in Sri Lanka (pp. 76-107).

Hettige, S. T. (1989). State monopolies and alcohol prevention - Sri Lanka. In T. Kortteinen (ed.), *State monopolies and alcohol prevention*. Helsinki: Social Research Institute of Alcohol Studies (pp. 559-579).

Hettige, S. T. (1990). Social research on alcohol in Sri Lanka: background issues and prospects. In J. Maula. et al. (eds.), *Alcohol in developing countries* (NAD Publication No. 18). Helsinki: Nordic Council for Drug Research (pp. 194-206).

Ministry of Health (1995, 2002). *Annual Health Bulletin*. Colombo: Department of Health Services.

National Dangerous Drug Control Board (1993). *Hand Book of Drug Abuse Information*. Colombo: National Dangerous Drug Control Board

Police Department (various years). *Administration Reports*. Colombo: Police Department.

Prisons Department (1995). *Prison Statistics*. Colombo: Prisons Department.

Ray, H.C. (ed., 1959). *History of Ceylon*. Colombo: University Press, University of Sri Lanka.

Registrar General's Office (various years). Vital Statistics Reports and unpublished data. Colombo: Department of Registrar General

Sarkar, N.K. (1957). *The demography of Ceylon*. Colombo: University of Ceylon, Government Press.

Sri Lanka Customs (various years up to 1996). *Annual Reports*. Colombo: Department of Customs.

CHAPTER 9

GENDER AND THE MAJOR CONSEQUENCES OF ALCOHOL CONSUMPTION IN UGANDA

NAZARIUS MBONA TUMWESIGYE & ROGERS KASIRYE

INTRODUCTION

INTRODUCTION

The republic of Uganda has a population of 23.8 million according to the 2002 census. It borders on Kenya to the east, Sudan to the north, Democratic Republic of Congo to the west, Tanzania to the south, and Rwanda to the extreme south west. Women constitute 51% of the population. The majority (85%) of the population is rural. As of 1991, half of the population was less than 17.2 years of age (Statistics Dept & MOFEP, 1995). The economy of the country is agricultural, with over 90% of the population dependent on subsistence farming and light agro-based industries.

Alcohol use, though not properly documented, is a widely accepted social activity. It is estimated that 5-10 % of the population is dependent on alcohol, and regular users experience alcohol related problems like ill health, marital disturbance and loss of employment (Jacobs, Aeron-Thomas, & Astropn, 2000). Use and abuse of alcohol is further facilitated by the fact that alcohol is quite often regarded as a social drink. It is used at cultural functions such as death, birth, marriage and circumcision ceremonies. Alcoholic beverages are therefore widely consumed by all people male and female, young and old with the exception of certain groups of people who are prohibited to drink due to religious and cultural reasons. Moslems and some reformed (born again) Christians are not allowed to drink alcohol, while women and children are culturally not allowed to drink in public.

Uganda lacks a clear alcohol policy. The commercial sale of traditionally produced spirits is regulated by the Liquor Licensing act of 1964 that forbids the sale and consumption of crude *Waragi* (local spirit). Such a law is outdated, weak and — worse still — not enforced. There is no law to regulate alcohol producers to prevent unfair advertising practices. Most advertising revenue in both print and electronic media and support to sports comes from the breweries. Consumption of factory beer is mainly urban, and brand switching at the individual level is limited by factors that include price, alcohol content, companion preferences, kind of entertainment, income level and advertising. The price of manufactured beer ranges from the equivalent of half a dollar for a large bottle upwards. There is low perception of risk of alcohol consumption (Willis, 2002). As a result of weak or non-existent policies on alcohol production, sale, marketing and consumption, the availability of alcohol, together with various social cultural and environmental factors, has created a situation of increased harmful and hazardous consumption of alcohol. Alcohol is known to be the most common substance of addiction used in the population. It is estimated that alcohol causes suffering to at least 70% of the population either directly or indirectly (Kigozi & Kasirye, 1997)

PRODUCTION OF ALCOHOL

The country is richly supplied with alcoholic beverages. There are many types of factory and locally brewed beer. Between 11 and 13 million crates of beer on average are produced in factories annually, contributing almost 10% of state revenue. There are also large amounts of informally produced alcoholic beverages which are unrecorded. It is these alcoholic beverages that are consumed by the majority of the population. Brewing and distilling of alcohol is also an accepted economic activity in the general population. In a study carried out in districts of Kabarole, Tororo and Gulu, it was found that drinking is central to the economy and social life of the family and community (Topouzis, 1994)

Many households in the country are involved in informal alcohol production at home, from which they get a substantial cash income. The money raised is used to pay school fees and for day-to-day home expenses. Although both men and women are engaged in production of different alcoholic drinks, the types made from grains are almost always made by women (Willis, 2002). There have not been major changes in the roles of men and women in making alcohol beverages over the years. However, there has been a change in drinking patterns, with more women drinking alcohol (Mulimbura, 1977). Consumption by women is affected by exposure through their involvement in the sale of alcohol. In some situations women use children to sell the home-brewed alcohol, and as a result these children begin drinking as early as 8 years (Mulimbura, 1977). Women's participation in alcohol production is due to poverty and lack of alternative income-generating activities.

CONSUMPTION

The Uganda Demographic and Health Survey (UDHS) found that one in four women and almost one in two men consumed alcohol at least once in the previous 30 days (UBOS & ORC Macro, 2001). Among those who drank, one in four women and one in two men got drunk at least once in that period. The increasing involvement of children in local alcohol production and sale is likely to raise their level of alcohol consumption. In general, children are still restricted in the amount of alcohol they can take and when to take it but this is difficult to monitor.

Research findings have attributed high alcohol consumption to political instability, poverty, unemployment and culture. Uganda's protracted war and political turmoil made people demoralized, lose interest in the future and resort to excessive drinking (Topouzis, 1994). Based on the findings, the current level of alcohol consumption should be high in the northern part of the country, where there is insecurity caused by a running rebellion and more poverty compared to the rest of the country.

Some researchers have suggested that poverty and related hardship might cause or increase the level of alcohol consumption while others suggest that the reverse is true. According to the 1999 Uganda participatory poverty assessment project (UPPAP), excessive drinking was among 5 major causes of poverty in the country (Lwanga-Ntale & Kimberly, 2003). In a study carried out in 1997, it was found that low economic productivity in the Kabale district was partly attributable to consumption of home-brewed alcohol (Puhalla, 2003).

Culture is also implicated in the high level of alcohol consumption in Uganda. In some cultural groups, when a child is given a name, it is also given alcohol to mark the occasion (Topouzis, 1994). Other occasions like circumcision, funeral rites and weddings cannot be complete without drinking alcohol. Inclusion of alcohol in the customs signifies the importance of alcohol in people's lives. Most times alcohol is taken frequently and in excessive quantities because people see it as part of their life. Other people see it as a duty one has to fulfil. Men who don't drink are often not respected; drinking is identified with virility. This makes alcohol an integral part of the whole village culture and a catalyst in social interaction, but also a distraction depending on time spent, cost and consequences of its consumption.

CONSEQUENCES

Research has shown that a history of alcohol consumption is associated with an increased chance of being infected with HIV. A study carried out in Uganda found that people who drank alcohol were twice as likely to be HIV-positive as abstainers (Mbulaiteye, Ruberantwari, Nakiyingi et al., 2000).

In families, alcohol dependence has been found to be a major problem that leads to broken homes (Mushanga, 1974). Alcohol consumption separates people, disrupts family unity and destroys marriage (NCC & GOU, 1994). Alcohol-dependent persons are more frequently divorced or separated than others, and their wives or husbands and children have relatively high rates of physical, emotional and psychosomatic illnesses (Mushanga, 1974).

Disability and deaths caused by alcohol-related traffic accidents are still unquantified in Uganda, and yet the country is rated fourth in the number of traffic accident deaths per 10,000 motor vehicles in Africa (Jacobs, Aeron-Thomas, & Astropn, 2000). The traffic law against drink driving was not adequately enforced by the police due to lack of equipment to test alcohol content in blood or breath. Alcohol has been shown to be a likely contributing factor in accidents in previous research (Kobusingye, Guwatudde, & Lett, 2001).

There is a high level of domestic violence in rural areas, and it has been linked to alcohol consumption and perceived risk of HIV. In a study by researchers from the Johns Hopkins Bloomberg School of Public Health, approximately one in three women living in rural Uganda reported being physically threatened or assaulted by their current partner. The findings from the study suggest possible links between the risk of domestic violence and alcohol consumption and women's perceived risk of contracting HIV from their partners (Koenig, Lutalo, Feng et al., 2003).

There is still a lot that is unknown about the levels of alcohol consumption and its associated problems and benefits in Uganda. The little research that has been done on alcohol consumption lacks national representativeness, is not detailed enough to cover all major issues on alcohol, and shows inconsistent results. In addition, the methods used are incapable of allowing precise estimates. For example the prevalence of alcohol dependence of 5-10% (Jacobs et al. 2000) and the proportion suffering (at least 70%) directly or indirectly as a result of alcohol consumption (Kigozi & Kasirye, 1997) are not estimated precisely enough, and the differences between estimates are large.

THE GENACIS PROJECT IN UGANDA

In 2003, Uganda was one of the countries that participated in the multinational project on Gender, Alcohol and Culture: an International Study (GENACIS). The study aimed at obtaining information on gender differences in consumption and drinking patterns, alcohol problems, experience of domestic violence, and at making comparisons between countries in relation to society-level variables. The objectives of this paper are to describe the patterns of alcohol consumption, establish factors associated with alcohol consumption, and determine the relationship between alcohol consumption and negative consequences measured.

METHOD

STUDY SETTING

The GENACIS study was designed as a cross-sectional quantitative study. It was carried out in the districts of Kabale, Wakiso, Tororo and Lira to represent the western, central, eastern and northern regions of Uganda, respectively. The respondents were men and women aged 18 years and above who were residents of the villages and towns they were found in at survey time.

Within each region, the selected district represented districts most likely to have alcohol-related problems. In the north, Lira has internally displaced persons, while in the west, Kabale is among the districts leading in alcohol-related crime. Illegal production and consumption of crude local spirits are at a high level in Kabale district. Most people in Lira, especially in the northern part of the district, moved towards the town due to insecurity caused by a rebellion against the government. In the central region, Wakiso is among the most urbanised, with high consumption of factory-brewed beer, while in the east, Tororo, being at the busiest border point, has had alcohol-related problems and drug abuse for many years.

RESEARCH INSTRUMENT

Few changes were made to a standard 30-page questionnaire from the World Health Organisation to reflect local context. The instrument was translated into local languages before being used for data collection. Education and urbanization levels were changed to suit the local classifications. Names, terms and sizes for different brands of home and factory-made alcohol were included, together with their alcohol content. All questions relating to forms of sexual orientation other than heterosexual were deleted because of fear of negative reactions they would cause. A question on sexual partners in the previous 12 months was changed to include sexual partners in the previous two years. Five questions on condom use were added in the intimate relations and sexuality section, primarily meant for those aged 18-24 years.

SAMPLING

The sex and age distribution of the total sample was nearly the same as in the national census. The Primary Sampling Units (PSUs) were sub-counties in the study districts and counties (all counties were visited). Secondary Sampling Units (SSUs) were parishes and Tertiary Sampling Units (TSUs) were villages. Lists of counties, sub-counties and parishes were obtained from the Uganda National Bureau of Statistics, while names of villages were obtained from local leaders at the parish level. The under-coverage included people living in inaccessible places such as on steep hills and in marshy lands, those in insecure areas and people who could not remember or be helped to remember their age. The government security personnel advised the study team on which villages were safe and unsafe.

Within each selected district, a mix of sampling techniques was used. For a start, there was stratification by county, and then 50% of the sub-counties and 25% of the parishes were selected by simple random sampling technique. Within each parish, one village was randomly selected. In each village, a random sample of 11 households was selected using systematic sampling. According to the technique, the data collectors moved to the centre of the village and spun a pen to obtain a direction by random. Every other household (one in two) in the selected direction was visited until the total was 11. In the event that the end of the village was reached before getting 11 households, the pen was spun again and a new direction taken. If two or more household members were more than 17 years old, a table of random numbers or folded numbered pieces of paper was used to select one by chance. The sample consisted of 1,479 respondents, with a response rate of 83.6%.

PROCEDURE

Prior to data collection, research assistants were selected through an interview and rigorously trained on both theory and practical aspects of data collection. One of the issues covered was ensuring confidentiality and creating a good environment in which the respondents would provide accurate data. In situations where respondents were in the company of other people, the advice was to seek permission to move with the respondent a few metres away from other people.

At the start of data collection, the research assistants were given a list of all types of drinks and the corresponding volumes that contained 12 grams of ethanol, used as a standard measure of a drink. The volumes were determined after a government chemist had measured the alcohol content of each beverage. Samples of the local drinks that were measured for alcoholic content were obtained from a Kampala city suburb. Nearly all alcoholic beverages made in rural homes are also made in urban centres to cater for low income earners who cannot afford factory made drinks. The survey was carried out using face-to-face interviews.

ANALYSIS

All data were entered in EPINFO 2000 and exported to STATA V.8E. The dependent variables of interest were frequency of drinking, quantity drunk and negative experiences thought to be associated with alcohol consumption. The experiences were quarrelling, having more than one sexual partner in the previous 2 years, physical aggression and smoking. For further analysis, frequency of alcohol consumption and quantity of alcohol were coded as binary outcome variables: having drunk alcohol at least three times a week, and taking 12 or more drinks in a single day in the previous 12 months. The explanatory variables were sex, age group, education level, income level, tribe, region, rural/urban residence, marital status, number of households in the family, feeling lonely, membership in a society, occupation, religion and the persons with whom the respondent was living.

In the first stage of analysis, the sample was described by distribution of key background characteristics. Cross-tabulation of demographic characteristics with quantity drunk and frequency of alcohol consumption was made to describe the level and patterns of alcohol consumption. The format of the cross-tabulations and the selection of variables were determined by the GENACIS research collaboration to allow comparability across countries.

The second stage of analysis involved determining the significance of the unadjusted effect of each independent variable on the outcome variables. The variables, which had a p-value of less than 0.2 in a log likelihood ratio test, were used to build a final multivariate model. Using a backward stepwise estimation method a final model was made with elimination criteria of 0.2. The models were tested for goodness of fit using the predictive power (proportion of rightly predicted), Lemeshow test, and specificity and sensitivity tests.

RESULTS

BACKGROUND CHARACTERISTICS

The distribution of respondents by district was 29% for Kabale, 21% for Lira, 25% for Tororo and 26% for Wakiso. Table 1 shows that the sample was composed of 49% men and 51% women. The male-female ratio was lowest in Kabale (1:1.5) and highest in Lira (1:0.5). Nearly half (47%) of the respondents were in the age group 18-29. The majority of respondents were from ethnic groups of Bakiga (27%), Baganda (20%), Langi (19%) and Adhola (19%).

Most respondents (86.8%) had received some kind of formal education, with 33.4% and 38.9% having attained primary and secondary education, respectively. A large proportion of respondents belonged to three major religions in the country. Nearly a half (48.1%) of the participants were Catholic, 33.3% were Protestant and 9.5% were Moslem. A half (50.5%) of the respondents lived in rural areas, 28.3% lived in suburbs and the rest in towns. Uganda is 85% rural, and the difference between this and the present sample results from a large number of people displaced into towns in northern Uganda due to insecurity. Another reason is the inclusion of the Wakiso district, which is among the most urbanised districts in the country.

More than half of the respondents (59.1%) were married. Major occupations were peasant farming (25.6%) and unskilled labour (26.3%). The majority were occupied as unskilled workers (26.3%) and smallholder farmers (25.6%). A fifth of the respondents earned the equivalent of less than US$ 225, while 40.8% earned between US$ 225 and US$ 900 a year. More than a half lived with their spouses (54%) or with their partners' under age children.

TABLE 1.   Background characteristics of respondents by district (%)

Characteristic	Kabale (n = 428)	Lira (n = 305)	Tororo (n = 365)	Wakiso (n = 381)	All (N=147)9	Uganda (1991 census)
Sex						
Male	43.5	65.9	47.4	42.3	48.8	49.1
Female	56.5	34.1	52.6	57.7	51.2	50.9
Age						
18-29	47.9	37.7	42.7	57.0	46.9	21.2
30-44	36.5	43.9	38.4	32.8	37.5	13.1
45+	15.7	18.4	18.9	10.2	15.6	12.0
Tribe						
Muganda	2.8	0	3.8	69.6	19.7	18.1
Mukiga	84.4	0.3	0	7.9	26.5	8.3
Adhola	0.2	1.0	56.4	0	14.2	1.5
Langi	0	89.2	0.6	0.5	18.7	5.9
Others	12.7	9.5	39.2	21.7	20.9	66.2
Education						
None	19.6	12.1	13.7	4.5	12.7	36.9
Primary	34.1	29.2	41.6	28.1	33.4	52.8
Secondary	33	36.1	37.6	49.1	38.9	8.7
Post secondary	12.9	22.3	7.1	17.4	14.6	0.3
Missing	0.47	0.3	0	1.1	0.5	1.3
Religion						
Moslem	4.4	8.2	7.4	18.1	9.5	10.5
Protestant	46.3	36.4	21.4	27.8	33.3	39.2
Catholic	44.6	50.8	60.3	38.1	48.1	44.5
Others	2.3	0	4.7	11.3	4.7	5.7
Missing	2.3	4.6	6.3	4.7	4.4	0.1
Residence						
Rural areas	60.7	36.7	73.2	28.1	50.5	85.3
Small town	1.4	14.4	3.6	22.1	9.9	-
Medium size town	15	16.1	14.0	0.8	11.3	-
In a suburb/trading centre	22.9	32.8	9.3	49.1	28.3	-
Marital status						
Never Married	30.4	26.6	17.5	39.1	28.7	41.8
Married/with partner	60.7	58	72.4	45.7	59.1	47.9
Other	8.4	15.5	9.9	15	11.9	10.0
Missing	0.5	0	0.27	0.3	0.3	0.3
Occupation						
Unskilled labour	24.1	26.9	23.6	31.0	26.3	-
Peasant farming	29.0	27.9	39.5	6.8	25.6	73.9
Technician/clerical	3.0	6.6	3.8	3.2	4.0	3.1
Professional	13.1	16.1	5.2	13.9	12.0	0.3
Homemaker	7.9	6.6	14.3	15.8	11.2	-
Small business	4.9	4.3	5.2	9.2	6.0	6.9
Student	14.2	9.2	6.3	13.7	11.0	-
Unemployed	2.1	1.6	1.4	6.0	2.8	-
Income						
Bottom quarter (<US$225)	27.8	17.7	28.2	5.0	20.0	-
Middle half (US$ 225-900)	34.1	44.3	35.3	50.9	40.8	-
Top quarter (US$>900)	14.3	19.7	7.7	30.7	18.0	-
Missing	23.8	18.4	28.8	13.4	21.2	-
Living with						
Spouse/partner	55.6	47.9	69.3	42.3	54.0	-
Partner's under age children	51.9	55.7	60.8	38.1	51.3	-
Partner's adult children	14.7	14.4	17.0	10.5	14.1	-
Partner's parents	8.6	7.2	7.7	1.6	6.3	-
Other relatives	28.5	32.5	29.6	46.7	34.3	-

PATTERN OF DRINKING

Of the total number of respondents, 47% reported that they drank alcohol, with men (55%) being more likely to drink than women (40%). A third of the respondents were lifelong abstainers, while a fifth had stopped drinking. Men were more likely (40.1%) to be long-time drinkers than women (23.5%) [See Table 2]. Lifetime abstention was less common among older groups of men and women and being an ex-drinker was more common with advancing age, at least among women. The difference by gender changed direction among new drinkers. A slightly higher percentage of young women (28%) than of young men (26.1%) were new drinkers. Among the middle aged (30-44) and the older (45+), men were more likely to drink for a longer time compared to women.

TABLE 2.   Pattern of drinking by gender and age group (%)

Drinking status	Men				Women				All
	18-29 (n = 314)	30-44 (n = 289)	45+ (n = 118)	All (n = 721)	18-29 (n = 379)	30-44 (n = 266)	45+ (n = 113)	All (n = 758)	(N = 1479)
Drank for > 10 years	14.3	57.4	66.1	40.1	8.7	38.4	38.1	23.5	31.6
Current drinker*	26.1	8.0	0	14.6	28.0	4.9	3.5	16.2	15.4
Former drinker	18.8	14.2	17.8	16.8	21.4	23.7	32.7	23.9	20.4
Life long abstainer	40.8	20.4	16.1	28.6	42.0	33.1	25.7	36.4	32.6

*Drank alcohol at study time but started within last 10 years

FREQUENCY OF DRINKING

Among the drinkers, a third drank nearly daily or more often. This implies that the proportion of daily drinkers was 15.5 %, since 47% drank alcohol at the time of the study. Table 3 shows that men were more than twice (44.7%) as likely to be daily drinkers as the women (17.6%). Nearly

TABLE 3.   Frequency of drinking (%)

Frequency	Men				Women				All
	18-29 (n =127)	30-44 (n =189)	45+ (n =78)	All (n = 394)	18-29 (n =139)	30-44 (n = 115)	45+ (n = 47)	All (n = 301)	(N = 695)
Less than monthly	20.5	10.6	6.4	12.9	41.7	40.9	25.5	38.9	24.2
Monthly	19.7	8.5	21.8	14.7	20.9	24.4	21.3	22.3	18.0
Weekly	24.4	34.4	16.7	27.7	21.6	17.4	29.8	21.3	24.9
Near daily	35.4	46.6	55.1	44.7	15.8	17.4	23.4	17.6	33.0

similar patterns are evident in all age groups. Daily drinking increased with age among men.

HIGHEST QUANTITY OF ALCOHOL TAKEN IN A SINGLE DAY IN PREVIOUS 12 MONTHS

Data in Table 4 show that of the respondents who drank alcohol, 14% had ever taken at least 12 drinks in a single day in the previous 12 months. (A drink was any amount and type of alcoholic beverage that contained 12 grams of ethanol). Men were nearly three times as likely as women to have taken at least 12 drinks in a day within the previous 12 months. Unlike the pattern for frequency of drinking, the pattern for drinking 12 or more drinks was for the middle-aged respondents to consume more than the younger and older groups among both women and men.

TABLE 4.   Highest quantity drunk in a single day in previous 12 months (%)

Quantity (Drinks)	Men				Women				All
	18-29 (n = 127)	30-44 (n = 189)	45+ (n = 78)	All (n = 394)	18-29 (n = 139)	30-44 (n = 115)	45+ (n = 47)	All (n = 301)	(N = 695)
<1	1.6	0.5	1.3	1.0	6.5	3.5	8.5	5.7	3.0
1-2	15.0	12.2	11.5	12.9	27.3	27.0	34.0	28.2	19.6
3-4	19.7	19.1	12.8	18.0	28.1	20.9	17.0	23.6	20.4
5-7	20.5	20.6	21.8	20.8	14.4	12.2	17.0	14.0	17.8
8-11	19.7	13.2	26.9	18.0	3.6	11.3	2.1	6.3	13.0
12+	17.3	23.8	14.1	19.8	5.0	10.4	4.3	7.0	14.2
Unknown*	6.3	10.6	11.5	9.4	15.1	14.8	17.0	15.3	11.9

* Respondent could not remember

A high proportion of men (75.7%) had taken a maximum of three or more drinks in a single day in the previous 12 months, with the commonest quantity being 5-7 drinks (20.8%). Among women, a lesser proportion (50.7%) had taken three or more drinks, and the most preferred (28%) quantity was 1-2 drinks.

FREQUENCY AND QUANTITY DRUNK

The respondents were classified into five categories depending on the frequency and quantity of alcohol they drink. These were abstainers, infrequent-light drinkers, frequent-light drinkers, infrequent-heavy drinkers and frequent-heavy drinkers. The abstainers included those who had never taken alcohol and those who were abstaining at the time of the study but had ever taken alcohol. Infrequent-light drinkers always drank less than 5 drinks on an occasion and drank less than 12 times in the previous 12 months. Frequent-light drinkers drank alcohol at least once a month, but without drinking as much as 5 drinks. Infrequent-heavy drinkers drank 5 or more drinks on some occasions, but drank less that 12 times in the previous 12 months. Frequent-heavy drinkers drank 5 or more drinks on an occasion and drank at least once a month in the previous 12 months.

Table 5 shows that men were more likely (22.9%) to be frequent heavy drinkers than women (6.5%). Heavy drinking increased with age among men, while it did not vary much among women. Whereas level of abstinence from alcohol reduced with age among men, it increased with age among women. Among the age group 18-29, there was not much difference by gender in the proportion of abstainers.

TABLE 5.   Typology of drinking (%)

Typology	Men				Women				All
	18-29 (n = 314)	30-44 (n = 289)	45+ (n = 118)	All (n = 721)	18-29 (n = 379)	30-44 (n = 266)	45+ (n = 113)	All (n = 758)	(N = 1479)
Abstainer	59.6	34.6	33.9	45.4	63.1	56.8	58.4	60.2	52.9
Infrequent light	4.5	6.9	5.1	5.6	11.1	11.3	8.0	10.7	3.2
Frequent light	9.6	13.8	12.7	11.8	11.9	10.9	15.0	12.0	11.9
Infrequent heavy	8.6	12.5	8.5	10.1	6.1	5.6	4.4	5.7	7.8
Frequent heavy	15.0	26.3	35.6	22.9	4.5	8.7	8.0	6.5	14.5
Missing	2.9	5.9	4.2	4.3	3.4	6.8	6.2	5.0	4.7

CONTEXTS OF DRINKING FOR CURRENT DRINKERS

Of the respondents who were current drinkers, most took it at parties (80.9%) or in bars (68.6%). The places or times when most respondents would rarely drink were workplaces (88.8%), during working hours (85.7%) and restaurants (77.5%). The men who drank in bars were more likely to be weekly clients (46.8%) compared to those who drank in other places, while among the women, it was those who drank at home that were more likely (20%) to drink weekly. As shown in Table 6, the most common companions for men when taking alcohol were friends and workmates, while for women they were friends and family members. Workmates were the second most common (31%) weekly companion for men, while for women it was spouses/partners (14.2%).

Two-thirds of the men drank during the evening on weekends, while a half drank during evenings on weekdays. A small proportion (3.3%) drank an hour before driving or during the day on weekdays (17.6%). A similar pattern was observed among the women.

TABLE 6. **Frequency of drinking alcohol with different companions (%)**

	MEN					WOMEN					All
	Never	Less than monthly	1-3 times a month	Weekly	N	Never	Less than monthly	1-3 times a month	Weekly	N	Never
With spouse /partner	47.0	29.6	9.7	13.7	372	42.9	31.2	11.7	14.2	282	45.3
With family member	36.4	38.0	9.0	16.5	387	41.8	42.8	5.7	9.7	299	38.8
With workmates	34.7	28.4	6.0	31.0	381	60.7	28.4	4.2	6.7	285	45.8
Friends	9.3	29.5	10.9	50.4	387	23.8	43.6	14.1	18.5	298	15.6
Alone	38.3	26.7	9.3	25.7	389	49.7	26.3	10.0	14.0	300	43.3

CONSEQUENCES OF ALCOHOL CONSUMPTION AMONG CURRENT DRINKERS

Table 7 shows that, overall, the most commonly reported consequences associated with alcohol consumption among current drinkers were financial problems (44%) and poor physical health (28.7%). The prevalence of the consequences was higher among men (finance, 56.4%; physical health 32.0%) than among women (finance, 27.9%; physical

TABLE 7. **Consequences of alcohol consumption (in percent of for current drinkers)**

Typology	Men				Women				All
	18-29 (n = 314)	30-44 (n = 289)	45+ (n = 118)	All (n = 721)	18-29 (n = 379)	30-44 (n = 266)	45+ (n = 113)	All (n = 758)	(N = 1479)
Harmed finances	57.7	57.1	52.6	56.4	23.7	27.7	40.4	27.9	44.0
Physical health	33.1	34.9	22.7	32.0	24.3	23.7	27.7	24.6	28.7
Harmed housework	17.6	24.6	17.1	20.9	20.9	21.2	25.5	21.7	21.3
Harmed work/study	24.0	27.8	19.7	25.0	14.6	15.3	15.9	15.0	20.7
Harmed Marriage	22.9	31.3	17.1	25.8	10.8	10.7	4.7	9.8	18.9
Had an injury /injured somebody	19.4	30.8	23.1	25.3	10.8	8.7	5.7	9.2	18.2
Harmed family relationship	20.2	26.2	17.1	22.5	7.9	11.5	10.6	9.7	16.9
Harmed friendship	21.8	21.8	13.2	20.1	10.7	8.0	10.6	9.7	15.6

health 24.6%). The most common personal experiences with alcohol were drinking-related illness (25.3%), and criticism from other people (25.2%). The least common experiences were losing a job (7.7%) and trouble with the law because of drunk driving (13.0%). Among men, it was the middle aged who were most likely to suffer the consequences, while among women it was those in the older age group.

Two thirds of all the drinkers (66%) had had a problem associated with alcohol consumption in their social life in the last 12 months. The problems which were thought to have occurred as a result of alcohol consumption were poor relationships with family members and other people, poor work/studies, fighting, law-breaking, financial difficulties and pressure from people to cut down on alcohol consumption. Table 8 shows that women were less likely (56%) to face social consequences of alcohol consumption than men (74%). Half of all the respondents had faced health consequences of alcohol consumption and men were 1.5 times more likely to face health consequences than women.

TABLE 8. **A score for all social and health consequences combined**

Consequences	Male (n=394)	Female (n=301)	Total (N=695)
Social			
None	26.1	44.5	34.1
One	11.4	13.0	12.1
Two	9.6	10.6	10.1
Three or more	52.8	31.9	43.7
Health			
None	43.9	59.1	50.5
One	26.9	21.6	24.6
Two	17.0	13.3	15.4
Three or more	12.2	6.0	9.5

QUARRELLING WITH SPOUSES/PARTNERS

Two-thirds of the respondents had ever quarrelled with their spouses/partners, while 32.7% had ever quarrelled with them after drinking alcohol. Among those who had ever quarrelled with their partners and were non-abstainers, 67% quarrelled after they had drunk alcohol. Men were more likely (75%) to quarrel with their spouse/partner after drinking alcohol than women (57%).

FACTORS ASSOCIATED WITH ALCOHOL CONSUMPTION

Multivariate models were built from bivariate analysis using background characteristics as independent variables and drinking three or more times a week as a dependent variable. The same style of analysis was carried out with having taken more than 12 drinks on a single day as the dependent variable. Another set of models examined the strength of association between frequent drinking (three or more times a week) and risky behaviour, smoking, experience of physical aggression and quarrelling with partner.

In Table 9, factors associated with frequent drinking in a multivariate model were found to be sex, age, religion, occupation and loneliness. A male aged 30 years and above, Christian, staying at home and not lonely was most likely to drink more frequently. Being at home could also mean working from home, including brewing beer, apart from referring to

TABLE 9. **Correlates of high frequency drinking (3 or more times a week) among current drinkers**

Variable	Bivariate		Multivariate[1]	
	OR	**95%CI**	**OR**	**95%CI**
Sex (Male=0/Female=1)	0.23**	0.17-0.32	0.19***	0.13-0.28
Age group				
18-29	1			
30-44	2.25**	1.62-3.13	1.79*	1.23-2.60
45+	2.85**	1.92-4.23	2.36***	1.51-3.70
Number of times lonely				
1-2	1			
3-4	0.73	0.54-1.00	0.69*	0.49-0.97
5-7	0.68	0.44-1.05	0.73	0.45-1.16
Member of a social support group (Yes=1/No=0)	0.80	0.59-1.06	--	
Religious preference				
Catholic	1.0			
Protestant	0.87	0.64-1.17	0.85	0.61-1.17
Moslem	0.19	0.08-0.44	0.18***	0.08-0.43
Daily Occupation				
Stay at home/homemaker	1			
Unemployed/retired/not working	0.82	0.42-1.60	0.44*	0.21-0.92
Students	0.63	0.34-1.16	0.36**	0.17-0.74
Working for a pay	1.25	0.83-1.89	0.55*	0.33-0.90
Self employed	1.25	0.84-1.86	0.55*	0.34-0.88
Goodness of fit	--	--		
Pseudo R^2			12.4%	
Lemeshow test	--	--	0.08	--
% Correctly predicted by model	--	--	83	--
Sensitivity/specificity (%)	--	--	2.7/99.7	--

[1]Variable selection criteria was $p=0.2$ * $p<0.05$ ** $p<0.01$ *** $p<0.005$

homemakers. Being less lonely could also mean that the person felt lonely several times but always looked for company. People aged 30+ were nearly twice as likely to drink frequently as the young (<30 years). Women were much less likely to drink frequently than men. Moslems were much less likely to be frequent drinkers than Catholics. The variables adjusted for in the multivariate models were age group, education level, tribe, region, rural/urban residence, marital status, number of households in the family, feeling lonely, membership in an association and religion.

Table 10 shows that factors associated with heavy drinking (drank 12 or more drinks a single day) were gender, region and number of living children. Men with 2-3 children alive were most likely to have drunk 12 or more units of alcohol in one day within the previous twelve months. Men were nearly three times as likely to drink 12 or more drinks a day as women. People in the northern region were twice as likely to be heavy drinkers as those in central region. Insecurity and displacement of people in the region might explain the high consumption of alcohol. In the eastern region people might drink less than in the central region because they had relatively less income to spend. As Table 10 shows, people with 2 to 3 children were more likely to drink 12 or more units than those with none or one child. The variables adjusted for in the multivariate model were age group, education level, tribe, region, rural/urban residence, marital status, number of households in the family, feeling lonely, membership in an association and religion.

TABLE 10. Correlates of heavy drinking (drank 12 or more drinks in a single day) among current drinkers

Variable	Bivariate		Multivariate[1]	
	OR	95%CI	OR	95%CI
Sex (Male=0/Female=1)	0.32***	0.19-0.53	0.36***	0.21-0.61
Region				
Central	1			
Western	1.49	0.81-2.74	1.45	0.77-2.74
Eastern	0.41	0.18-0.96	0.39*	0.16-0.91
Northern	2.56*	1.32-4.93	2.03*	1.02-4.04
Number of Children alive				
0-1	1			
2-3	2.75*	1.36-5.57	3.07**	1.45-6.48
4/5	1.46	0.83-2.56	1.51	0.84-2.71
6+	1.2	0.69-2.10	1.27	0.71-2.28
Goodness of fit				
Lemeshow test	--	--	0.10	--
% Correctly predicted by model	--	--	84	--
Sensitivity/Specificity (%)	--	--	3/99.6	--

[1]Variable selection criteria was $p=0.2$ * $p<0.05$ ** $p<0.01$ *** $p<0.005$

Association of alcohol with negative outcomes

Frequent drinking featured as a strong correlate of quarrelling, having more than one sexual partner, experience of physical aggression and smoking in bivariate and multivariate models, after controlling for background information. People who drank at least three times a week were 1.6 times more likely to have quarrels with their partners than those who didn't. The results in Table 11 show that they were 1.5 times more likely to have more than 1 sexual partner, 1.9 times more likely to experience physical aggression and 5 times more likely to smoke. A test of interaction between frequency of drinking and gender was not statistically significant in the models for risky behaviour (II), physical aggression (III) and smoking (IV). This implies that relations with frequent drinking did not significantly vary by gender. The interaction was not tested in the quarrelling model (Model I) because gender was not a significant factor. Compared to other models, model I (quarrelling) had the least number of significant control variables and the predictive power was the lowest. This shows that there could be other factors confounding the relationship between frequency of drinking and quarrelling. The variables adjusted for in the multivariate model were age group, education level, tribe, region, rural/urban residence, marital status, number of households in the family, feeling lonely, membership to a society and religion.

TABLE 11. **Influence of alcohol on negative experiences and risky behaviour among current drinkers**

Variable	Multivariate Models[1]			
	Quarrelling with partner	Having more than 1 sexual partner in past 2yrs	Physical aggression	Smoking
	Model 1	Model II	Model III	Model IV
Drinks at least 3 times a week	1.63** (1.15-2.31)	1.53* (1.06-2.21)	1.88*** 1.28-2.74	4.93*** (3.44-7.07)
Sex	NS	***	***	***
Age group	NS	*	**	**
Education	NS	NS	*	*
Region	*	*	*	NS
Residence	NS	**	NS	NS
Marital status	NS	*	***	NS
No of people live with	**	*	NS	*
Occupation	NS	*	NS	NS
Number of times lonely	NS	*	NS	NS
Religious affiliation	NS	NS	*	NS
Goodness of fit				
Lemeshow test	0.65	0.11	0.22	0.53
% Correctly predicted by model	66%	74%	81%	86%
Sensitivity/ specificity	95%/12%	31.6%/90.4	3.1%/99.6%	28%/97%

[1] Variable selection criteria was $p=0.2$ NS= $p>0.05$ * $p<0.05$ ** $p<0.01$ *** $p<0.005$

DISCUSSION

The results above show that nearly half of the respondents drank alcohol. Men were more likely (40%) to be long time drinkers than women (24%). A third of the respondents drank alcohol nearly daily. Forty five percent of males and a third of the females drank daily. Of those who drank, 14 % had ever taken at least 12 drinks a day. Alcohol was mostly taken at parties (81%) or in bars (69%). People rarely drank alcohol at work places, during working hours and in restaurants. Common consequences associated with alcohol were financial problems and poor physical health. Two-thirds of the current drinkers had a problem associated with alcohol in their social life. The factors associated with frequent alcohol consumption were being male, of older age (30+ years) and Christian; staying at home and being social. The factors associated with heavy drinking were being male, hailing from the northern and eastern regions and having 2-3 children. Frequent drinking of alcohol was independently associated with quarrelling with partner, having more than one sexual partner, physical aggression and smoking.

It is not surprising that nearly half (47%) of the respondents drank alcohol, given its strong cultural, social and economic links (Willis, 2002). Men, as expected, were more long time drinkers and at the same time more frequent and heavy drinkers compared to women. What is new in the patterns of drinking is that among young people, women were more likely to be current drinkers than men. This is a sign that women might be changing the traditional pattern of alcohol consumption; this is supported by earlier findings (Mulimbura, 1977).

Gender differences in drinking patterns in this study are not surprising. Results from similar GENACIS surveys show that men persist in drinking (and drinking heavily) longer in life than women (Hao, Zhonhua, Binglun et al., 2004; Kemm, 2003; Breslow & Smothers, 2004), and changes in traditional drinking patterns are most likely among the youngest and newest drinkers (Mateos, Paramo, Carrera et al., 2002; Suggs, 2001; Suggs, 1996; Plant, Miller, Thornton et al., 2000; Mateos, Paramo, Carrera et al., 2002)

The older generation seems to drink more heavily compared to other age groups. Probably this reflects a mix of reasons. Factors such as stress (Chittick 1958), inability to cope with the prevailing situation (Howard 1963), and socio-economic problems (Topouzis, 1994) may all apply in this circumstance. Stress may be due to several reasons including poor health among the older age group, poor care and loss of loved ones, especially children who leave behind orphans. Uganda has an estimated 2 million orphans, mainly due to AIDS. Economic hardships prevailing in the country, low prices for produce and a high unemployment level could also be associated with drinking by older people.

The results further show that although the older age group drank more frequently and in higher amounts, the middle age group was more likely to drink the largest amount at a single time. Cultural factors contribute to the high frequency of drinking. The role of culture is clear in findings of Topouzis (1994) and Barton & Wamai (1994). If drinking alcohol is an integral part of the village culture, a catalyst in social interaction and a duty one has to fulfil, then it is not surprising that some people drink everyday.

The findings show that there is a high rate of abstention in young men compared with middle aged and older men. This could be attributed to new movements within the Protestant and Catholic churches that discourage alcohol consumption and mainly target the youth. Another factor is lack of money to spend on alcohol. Many of the young men are either in school or do not have proper employment from which they can get money to spend on alcohol.

A party was the most common drinking environment. This might be due to the cultural influence which encourages the hosting of parties. It is an obligation to give a party at some time and to attend parties. Bars were the second most common environment for drinking, but not for women. This could mainly be due to cultural reasons (Willis, 2002). Traditionally men drank to interact with other men and discuss social and cultural matters in their villages (Topouzis, 1994). This is consistent with what is reported by several psychologists: that men do most of their drinking away from home while the women drink with their spouses and family members (Miller & Cervantes, 1998). Women sought other women to discuss issues that concerned them. It was a rare occurrence to find men drinking with their partners. Another explanation could be that drinking alcohol is not an activity that people always have to plan for, so that one invites family members. One is likely to drink with workmates because a decision to drink is made while with them during working hours. The most common drinking time is evening and weekend in Uganda. This is evident in both urban and rural areas.

Harm to one's finances, poor health and loss of relationships were but a few of the common consequences of alcohol. This is in agreement with other authors (Puhalla, 2003, Koenig et al., 2003, Opunyo,1998, and Mushanga, 1974). The prevalences of social (66%) and health consequences (50%) among current drinkers were high, the most common consequences of alcohol consumption being psychological harm and marriage problems. The proportion of people who quarrel after drinking was high, probably due to loss of self-restraint after drinking alcohol. In addition, the high prevalence of quarrelling is not surprising since the frequency of alcohol consumption is high especially among men (45% daily). In most cases of quarrelling, women tended to be the victims (Holmila, 1995).

The study showed that, apart from quarrelling, frequent drinking is associated with having more than one sexual partner, smoking and partner and physical aggression. This is in agreement with findings by Koenig and others (Koenig, Lutalo, Feng et al., 2003) that alcohol consumption reduces self-control over emotions and sexual behaviour. Several other studies have found similar links.

LIMITATIONS AND RECOMMENDATIONS

The study had its share of limitations. For example, the sample was not fully representative of the regions and districts covered. People who could not know their age or lived in inaccessible areas were excluded, and this might have caused a bias. Also some questions required recall of events over a long time. An example is drinking 12 or more drinks in a single occasion over the previous 12 months. Many people may not easily recall such event.

Seasonality may have had an effect on the amount drunk and frequency of drinking. During the rainy season people could be drinking more because they stayed indoors for longer periods of time. They could also drink less because they did not move a lot to work for money. This research was not able to investigate the seasonality effect.

The alcoholic contents of the home brewed beer varies from area to area. This study measured the content of the home brew in Kampala. The inclusion of key questions on alcohol consumption, its problems and consequences in major national surveys such as Uganda Demographic and Health Survey (UDHS) and National Household Survey (NHS) could increase knowledge on alcohol consumption levels, patterns and associated factors and problems. In addition, more studies would allow monitoring of the levels and patterns of alcohol consumption and associated problems.

There is enough evidence to evoke action against uncontrolled alcohol consumption in Uganda. The proportion of people experiencing negative health and social consequences of alcohol consumption is too high to ignore. The results of this analysis of the Uganda GENACIS data stress the need for increased support for people who are displaced in Lira district. This is a social wellbeing as well as a public health challenge for all involved in providing services to women, children and youth in the country as a whole.

REFERENCES

Breslow, R. A., & Smothers, B. (2004). Drinking patterns of older Americans: National Health Interview surveys, 1997-2001. *Journal of Studies on Alcohol,* **65**, 232-240.

Hao, W., Zhonhua, S., Binglun, L., Zhang, K., Yang, H., Chen, S. et al. (2004). Drinking and drinking patterns and health systems in the general population of five areas of China. *Alcohol and Alcoholism, 39*, 43-52.

Holmila, M. (1995). Alcohol and harm in the family. *Paper presented on at the European Conference on Health Society and Alcohol Paris, 12-14 December.*Copenhagen: WHO Regional Office for Europe (Euro/ICP/ALDT 94 03 /CN 01/29)

Jacobs, G., Aeron-Thomas, A., & Astropn, A. (2000). *Estimating global road fatalities* (Rep. No. 445). Crowthorne, UK: Transport Research Laboratory.

Kemm, J. (2003). An analysis by birth cohort of alcohol consumption by adults in Great Britain 1978-1998. *Alcohol and Alcoholism,* **2**, 147.

Kigozi, F., & Kasirye, R. (1997). *Alcohol, drug abuse and HIV AIDS in Uganda* Kampala, Uganda: Uganda AIDS Commission.

Kobusingye, O., Guwatudde, D., & Lett, R. (2001). Injury patterns in rural and urban Uganda. *Injury Prevention, 7,* 46-50.

Koenig, A. M., Lutalo, T., Feng, Z., Nalugoda, F., Wabwire-Mangen, F., Kiwanuka, N. et al. (2003). Domestic violence in rural Uganda: evidence from a community-based study. *Bulletin of the World Health Organization,* **81**, 53-60.

Lwanga-Ntale, C., & Kimberly, M (2003, July). Face of chronic poverty in Uganda as seen by the poor themselves. *Conference paper on Chronic and Development Policy, University of Manchester, 7 to 9 April 2003.* Development Research and Training (DRT), Kampala, Uganda

Mateos, R., Paramo, M., Carrera, I., & Rodriguez-Lopez, A. (2002). Alcohol consumption in a Southern European region (Galicia, Spain). *Substance Use and Misuse,* **37**, 1957-1976.

Mbulaiteye, S. M., Ruberantwari, A., Nakiyingi, J., Carpenter, L., Kamali, A., & Whitworth, J. (2000). Alcohol and HIV a study among sexually active adults in rural southwest Uganda. *International Journal of Epidemiology,* **29**, 911-915.

Miller, R. W., & Cervantes, A. E. (1998). Gender and patterns of alcohol problems: Pretreatment responses of women and men to the comprehensive drinker profile. *Journal of Clinical Psychology,* **53**, 263-277.

Mulimbura (1977). *Alcohol consumption in Uganda.* Bachelor of Arts Makerere University, Uganda.

Mushanga, T. M. (1974). *Criminal homicide in Uganda.* Nairobi: East African Literature Bureau.

NCC & GOU (1994). *Equity and vulnerability: a situation of women, adolescents and children in Uganda.* Kampala: Government of Uganda, Uganda National Council of Science and Technology.

Plant, M. L., Miller, P., Thornton, C., Plant, M. A., & Bloomfield, K. (2000). Life stage, alcohol consumption patterns, alcohol-related consequences and gender. *Substance Abuse,* **21**, 265-281.

Puhalla, J. M. (2003). *Soil fertility management by women farmers in Kabale district, Uganda,* Tallahassee: Department of Geography, University of Florida.

Statistics Dept & MOFEP (1995). *The 1991 Population and Housing Census: Analytical report, Demographic characteristics* Entebbe: Statistics Department.

Suggs, D. N. (1996). Mosadi Tshwene: the construction of gender and the consumption of alcohol in Botswana. *American Ethnologist,* **23**, 597-610.

Suggs, D. N. (2001). 'These young chaps think they are just men, too': redistributing masculinity in Kgatleng bars. *Social Science and Medicine,* **53**, 241-250.

Topouzis, D. (1994). *The socio-economic impact of HIV/AIDS on rural families with an emphasis on youth in Uganda.* (Rep. No. TCP/UGA/2256). Kampala, Uganda: Food and Agriculture Organisation of the United Nations (FAO).

UBOS & ORC Macro (2001). *Uganda Demographic and Health Survey 2000-2001.* Calverton, Maryland, USA: Uganda Bureau of Statistics and ORC Macro.

Willis, J. (2002). *Potent Brews: A Social History of Alcohol in East Africa, 1850-1999.* Oxford: James Curry Publishers.

CHAPTER 10

PROBLEMS FROM WOMEN'S AND MEN'S DRINKING IN EIGHT DEVELOPING COUNTRIES

ROBIN ROOM & KLARA HRADILOVA SELIN

The previous chapters in this monograph have examined specific aspects of drinking patterns, contexts and problems, as revealed by surveys linked with the GENACIS project, in each of eight developing societies. The present chapter is a first effort to analyze the data from the different surveys in a common frame. Our focus is on the respondents' reports of problems related to their own drinking.

On the one hand, there are obvious limits to this perspective. The drinker's view of problems may not coincide with the views of others around the drinker, including those who experience adverse effects from the drinking. Reports from surveys of household populations are also more likely to pick up less serious problems from drinking, missing really serious problems, since the latter are too infrequent to be accurately measured with the usual-sized population survey, and are often more frequent in the part of the population living outside regular households.

But, on the other hand, the perspective gives us a picture of an important part of the full spectrum of alcohol problems which is not measured in the usual health or social statistics. The estimates of alcohol's role in the Global Burden of Disease made as part of a Comparative Risk Analysis (Rehm et al., 2004) – discussed in the introductory chapter of this monograph – focus only on problems measured in death or morbidity statistics: illnesses or

---

Box 1. Drinking problem items analyzed in this chapter

During the last 12 months, ...
1. has your drinking had a harmful effect on your marriage or intimate relationships?
2. has your drinking had a harmful effect on your relationships with other family members, including your children?
3. has your drinking had a harmful effect on your friendships or social life?
4. have you gotten in a fight while drinking?
5. have you had trouble with the law about your drinking and driving?
6. has your drinking had a harmful effect on your work, studies or employment opportunities?
7. has your drinking had a harmful effect on your housework or chores around the house?
8. has your drinking had a harmful effect on your finances?
9. has your drinking had a harmful effect on your physical health?
10. have you had a feeling of guilt or remorse after drinking?

casualties. Missing from such analyses is the whole range of social problems from drinking, including problems in the family, in work life or similar roles, and in civil life and public order. There have been previous efforts to analyze survey data on these issues in developing countries (e.g., Demers et al., 2001). But the GENACIS studies differ in an important way from such efforts. Particularly for most of the developing countries included in GENACIS, a common questionnaire was used in each country, allowing a comparative analysis across different societies. The items included in the present analysis (Box 1) provide a wide coverage across different elements of social problems with drinking, along with one item on health problems. Included in them are two items concerning family roles, an item on friendship roles, two items about civil comportment, two items on job or home productive activities, an item on finances, and an item on physical health. Besides these nine items concerning tangible consequences of drinking, we have included for comparison with them an item about the respondent's feelings of guilt or remorse after drinking, as a first step in comparing the extent of internalization of negative feelings about problematic drinking in different cultural circumstances.

The approach taken in this chapter is to examine respondents' reports of problems from their own drinking in the samples from eight countries represented in this monograph. Fewer results are reported for Mexico, since the study there was done before the inception of the GENACIS project, and only 2 of the 10 items considered here were included in the Mexican questionnaire. The reader is referred to the previous chapters for details on the fieldwork in each country. We would note here only that the samples, while of defined general adult populations, generally represent a geographical area which is less than the whole country. The Brazilian sample, in particular, represents a limited area that is more middle-class than the country as a whole. While for convenience we use the name of the country for each sample, it should be kept in mind that the samples are not representative of the whole country.

Both because of this and because of the vagaries of meaning as items are translated into different languages, we pay limited attention here to the absolute levels of positive responses to the different items. More reliable, we feel, are the comparisons, in particular by gender and age, within each sample: those answering a question in a particular language and culture are more likely to be interpreting it in the same way. Given this approach to the analysis, we have used unweighted data in the analysis (although weighting the data where appropriate would not substantially change the results). The analysis is limited to those aged 18-65 in each sample.

THE NATIONAL CONTEXTS: DRINKING LEVELS AND PATTERNS AND POLICY RESPONSES

Before considering the results of the survey data, it is worth considering and comparing the national contexts with respect to alcohol consumption and policies. Table 1 shows consumption data drawn from the WHO Global Alcohol Database, as it was used in the Comparative Risk Analysis (Rehm et al., 2004), and data on alcohol policies in the eight countries collected for a recent WHO report (WHO, 2004). The countries are ordered in Table 1 in descending order on the Human Development Index (see Table 4 of the first chapter). This ordering places the four Latin American countries at the top, the two south Asian countries next, and the two African countries at the bottom.

It will be seen from Table 1 that, even in this selection of just 8 countries, there is no straightforward relationship between level of development and per-adult consumption (that is, litres per annum of pure ethanol per inhabitant aged 15 or over, including estimated unrecorded consumption).

TABLE 1. **Level and pattern of drinking, and status on selected alcohol control policies, in 8 developing countries, early 2000s**

Country	Per adult consumption	Pattern (4 = worse)	Age limit	# time & place restrictions	License for off-sale spirits	Beer /cola price	Spirits relative price	Advertising restrictions score	BAL & RBT
Argentina	16.30	2	18	6	Lic	3.29	20.01	6	0.5x
Costa Rica	6.70	4*	18	12	Lic	0.80	13.17	6	0.49x
Mexico	8.15	4	18	9	Lic	2.13	22.63	1fi	0.8x
Brazil	8.59	3	18	0	No	2.26	9.42	1	0.6~
Sri Lanka	0.57	3	18	9	Lic	1.37	34.05	3	0.6x
India	2.00	3	18	12	Lic	1.32	55.62	12	0.3~
Uganda	13.30	3	18	0	-	1.45	33.54	0	0.8~
Nigeria	6.94	2	18	6	Lic	2.33	84.07	3	0.0~

* Costa Rica is shown with a pattern score of 4 (twice) and 3 (once) in Rehm et al. (2004).

Per adult consumption: Rehm et al., 2004: Estimated ethanol consumption per person aged 15+ in 2000, in litres, including estimated unregistered consumption.

Drinking pattern: Rehm et al., 2004: hazardous drinking score (range 1 - 4, with 4 most hazardous), in principle a comparative score of the trouble expected per litre of alcohol. Based on survey data and/or expert judgement on 6 items, reflecting predominance of intoxication in drinking occasions (4 indicators), extent of drinking in public, frequency of drinking with meals (reverse scored).

Age limit: WHO, 2004:33: highest age limit for purchasing alcohol beverages (usually for spirits consumed on-premises, if limits vary); No = no age limit.

Time and place restrictions: WHO, 2004:27-28: a score (range 0 - 12) of how many of the following restrictions existed for each of beer, wine, spirits: restrictions of hours of sale; of days of sale; of places of sale; of density of outlets.

License for off-sale spirits: WHO, 2004:21-23: Lic = off-sale retail of spirits is specifically licensed; No = it is not.

Beer/cola price: WHO, 2004:44: ratio: price of an average bottle or can of beer/price of a soft drink of the same size, for off-premises consumption.

Spirits relative price: WHO, 2004:46-47: price ratio of an average 750 ml. bottle of spirits to the GDP per capita, multiplied by 10,000.

Advertising Restrictions score: WHO, 2004:65-66: one point for a ban on each of beer, wine, spirits on national TV, national radio, print media, billboards (range = 0 - 12). Half point for voluntary agreements or partial legal restrictions.

BAL level and RBT: WHO, 2004:37. The Blood Alcohol Level limit for driving an automobile, per mille (grams per litre), and whether Random Breath Testing is used to enforce this often (xx), sometimes (x), or rarely or never (~).

Argentina, near the top of the list, and Uganda, near the bottom, have the highest estimated consumption levels, putting Uganda as well as Argentina up at the level of southern European wine cultures and some European beer-drinking countries. On the other hand, estimated consumption in India, and particularly in Sri Lanka, is very low by global standards.

The second column of Table 1 shows each country's score on a hazardous drinking pattern score developed in the WHO Comparative Risk Analysis (Rehm et al., 2004). This score, which ranges from 1 (for the least hazardous pattern) to 4 (for the most hazardous), in principle measures the relative increase in adverse consequences to be expected from each extra litre of alcohol consumed. It is thus a separate dimension from level of consumption, and is designed to express cultural differences in drinking patterns which would affect the rates of casualties and other consequences from a given level of drinking. The score was derived from expert judgements and (where available) survey data on six dimensions of drinking patterns connected to increased hazard: high quantity per occasion, proportions of drinking to intoxication and rates of drinking in public places, the occurrence of fiesta drinking, and low proportions of daily drinking and drinking with meals (Rehm et al., 2001). The average level of the eight countries on the hazardous drinking score is about 3, which is about what would be expected for a sample of developing countries. Mexico and Costa Rica (the latter in some versions of the score) have been assigned higher scores than the average, and Argentina and Nigeria lower scores.

The remaining columns of Table 1 show the status of each country in the early 2000s on a range of indicators of alcohol policy. Uniformly, the 8 countries are reported to have a minimum drinking age of 18 for all alcoholic beverages, in the middle of the range of such ages internationally. There is considerable variation between the countries in the extent of reported time and place restrictions on sale of alcohol, with Brazil and Uganda having the fewest such restrictions and Costa Rica and India the most. Brazil is reported to have no specific licensing for alcohol sales, and the data for Uganda is lacking; the other 6 countries have some form of alcohol licensing, and Costa Rica also has a spirits production monopoly.

The "Beer/cola price" column is the ratio of the reported prices of an average bottle or can of beer and of a soft drink of the same size. A high ratio may reflect high beer taxes, or relatively high production costs or profits of breweries. The ratio is not related in any obvious way to the standard of living. Thus the highest ratio (Argentina) and the lowest (Costa Rica) are for the two highest-ranking countries in terms of the HDI. Costa Rica is apparently among the minority of countries where a beer is cheaper than a soft drink. The next column, the "spirits relative price", compares the price of a bottle of spirits with the Gross Domestic Product per capita. This index is affected by the standard of living, more indeed than by the level of spirits taxes, so that poorer countries tend to show a higher relative price. However, this does reflect the reality that a bottle of spirits is a greater luxury for the poor than for the affluent. Brazil and Costa Rica stand out on this index as having relatively low spirits prices.

The density of restrictions on alcohol advertising varies across the complete range in the sample of 8 countries. As for restrictions on sale, Uganda and Brazil are at the bottom on this indicator, joined by Mexico, with India clearly at the top. There is also a considerable range on the legal blood-alcohol limit for driving, with Nigeria and India showing the most stringent restrictions, and Uganda and Mexico the least. None of the countries reports strong enforcement of the limit, with random breath-testing done often. Brazil, India, Uganda and Nigeria report the least level of enforcement.

CURRENT DRINKING BY GENDER AND AGE

A precondition to the occurrence of problems related to one's own drinking is that one drinks at all. It is clear that abstention is much more common in much of the developing world than, say, in Europe – and that globally the proportion of abstainers is the most important determinant of differences in per-adult consumption. Variations between different global subregions in the amount of drinking per drinker (that is, with abstainers removed from the base) are an order of magnitude less than variations on a per-adult basis (Room et al., 2002; Babor et al., 2003).

Previous work has shown that both gender and age-norms on drinking at all differ greatly in different countries (e.g., Roizen, 1988; Room et al., 2002: 85, 97-98). Table 2 shows that, at the level of the behaviour of drinking at all, there are substantial differences in the eight countries in the present analysis. Drinking remains an uncommon behaviour among women in India and Sri Lanka, at whatever age. A bare majority of Sri Lankan men have had an alcoholic drink sometime in the last year, with little differentiation by age. Only a minority of Indian men have had a drink with those in the 30-49 age group more likely to be drinkers than younger or older men. At the other end of the spectrum, Argentina conforms to the western European pattern of near-universal drinking, though even here the drinking rate falls off with age among women. In all the other countries in the study, drinking is a minority behaviour among women aged 50 and over. But in Uganda and Brazil women in this age group are nevertheless more likely to drink than younger women. Both Uganda and Nigeria show a pattern, found elsewhere in Africa too (Roizen, 1988), of a lower rate of drinking among adults under age 30 than among older adults.

In terms of the further analyses in this paper, one caution from these findings is that the base numbers of drinkers are low among Indian and particularly Sri Lankan women, so that the results shown should be treated with considerable caution.

TABLE 2.   Percentage current drinkers (within the last 12 months) among those aged 18-65 in eight developing countries, by age and gender, GENACIS surveys

Age	Argentina	Costa Rica	Mexico	Brazil	Sri Lanka	India	Uganda	Nigeria
			MALES (in percent)					
<30	96	78	78	65	51	29	37	30
30-49	88	66	79	60	63	42	62	46
50+	93	58	68	56	52	24	68	45
			FEMALES (in percent)					
<30	88	51	45	42	7	5	36	14
30-49	75	42	48	32	7	6	43	26
50+	70	37	36	47	5	7	46	29
			MALE base Ns					
<30	133	153	1010	121	150	731	314	265
30-49	176	167	1003	175	250	586	324	583
50+	92	64	369	123	151	170	66	249
			FEMALE base Ns					
<30	150	250	1372	175	154	717	379	342
30-49	268	402	1476	209	285	579	476	476
50+	180	126	481	137	122	149	131	131

PROBLEMS FROM ONE'S OWN DRINKING, BY GENDER

Table 3 shows the percentages of male and female current drinkers reporting having experienced each of the 10 items detailed in Box 1 in the last 12 months. The stand-out in terms of rates reported is Uganda, with higher rates than any other country for 8 of the 10 items among men and 7 among women. The rates are sufficiently high to raise some question about what Ugandan respondents meant by their answers. However, it is worth noting that Uganda stands out in Table 1 also in terms of both a high estimated per-capita consumption and a relatively high hazardous drinking score.

At the other end of the spectrum, both male and female drinkers generally report low rates of problems in Argentina and Sri Lanka (except for "harmed finances" among Sri Lankan males).

Generally, male drinkers report a higher rate of a particular item than female drinkers, although the rates by gender are much more equal in Nigeria. It is notable that even for the item "has your drinking had a harmful effect on your housework or chores around the house?", which was added to the GENACIS questionnaire with women in mind, the male rate is generally at least as high as the female.

The differences between societies on some items are quite remarkable. Among men, there is substantial variation in response to the item, "have you gotten into a fight while drinking?", although it is a quite concrete item

TABLE 3. Percentage of current drinkers reporting 10 problems from their own drinking, among those aged 18-65 in eight developing countries, by gender, Genacis surveys

Problems	Argentina	Costa Rica	Mexico	Brazil*	Sri Lanka	India	Uganda	Nigeria
MALE DRINKERS								
(Base Ns)	(367)	(269)	(1833)	(251)	(312)	(496)	(384)	(457)
1. harmed marriage/intimate relations	8	16	-	7	2	14	27	9
2. harmed family relations	7	12	-	6	2	10	25	7
3. harmed friendships	4	6	-	4	2	13	21	9
4. fight while drinking	8	23	7	11	-	16	18	3
5. drink-driving	1	6	-	4	1	4	9	2
6. harmed work	4	8	1	5	7	11	28	10
7. harmed chores	1	5	-	6	6	14	23	9
8. harmed finances	5	21	-	7	25	34	59	19
9. harmed physical health	7	16	-	8	9	20	34	12
10. guilt/remorse	7	8	-	12	12	32	17	8
FEMALE DRINKERS								
(Base Ns)	(441)	(354)	(1406)	(201)	(38)	(84)	(297)	(211)
1. harmed marriage/intimate relations	0	2	-	4	0	4	9	11
2. harmed family relations	2	7	-	3	0	10	9	5
3. harmed friendships	1	2	-	2	3	7	10	11
4. fight while drinking	2	7	1	3	-	4	6	5
5. drink-driving	0	0	-	0	0	2	4	2
6. harmed work	0	2	0	2	3	4	14	7
7. harmed chores	1	3	-	3	5	6	22	9
8. harmed finances	0	6	-	3	3	21	28	18
9. harmed phys. health	2	9	-	2	6	10	26	12
10. guilt/remorse	1	2	-	11	0	16	13	4

* Only a 40% subsample were asked items 4, 5 and 10 in Brazil.

where variations in interpretation should be minor. Costa Rican, Ugandan and Indian men stand out on this item, perhaps offering some validation to the relatively high hazardous drinking scores (Table 1) for these societies. The item on drinking having a harmful effect on finances takes a

215

prominent position among the problem items particularly for the societies at the lower end of the HDI rankings (India, Uganda and Nigeria for both genders; Sri Lanka for men), although one-fifth of Costa Rican male drinkers also acknowledge this item.

PROBLEM SCORES BY GENDER AND BY GUILT

In Table 4, we first show for each gender a problems score — the average percentage reporting "yes" to each of the first 9 items in Box 1 – on a base of the current drinkers. For both men and women, Ugandan drinkers are more likely to report alcohol problems than drinkers elsewhere, with over 1/5 of the men and over 1/10 of the women answering "yes" per item. Among men, Indian and Costa Rican drinkers have the highest score, with the rate among Nigerian drinkers also somewhat exceeding that in the other societies. Among women, it is Nigerian drinkers who rank second, with a problems score rate equal to that of Nigerian male drinkers, and the small fraction of Indian women who drink at all ranks third.

The next row for each gender shows the same score computed on a base which includes all abstainers (scored 0 on the problems score). As can be seen in the last two rows of the table, the greater proportion of

TABLE 4. Problem scores among current drinkers and among adults and guilt/problem ratio, by gender, and gender ratios on drinking problem rates for drinkers and for adults, among those aged 18-65 in seven developing countries, GENACIS surveys

Problems	Argentina	Costa Rica	Brazil	Sri Lanka	India	Uganda	Nigeria
MALES							
Problems score (mean %/item), current drinkers	5.0	12.6	6.4	6.8	12.8	22.0	8.9
Problems score, all adults	4.7	8.7	3.8	3.9	4.2	11.2	3.7
Guilt/problem ratio	1.4	0.6	1.9	1.8	2.5	0.8	0.9
FEMALES							
Problems score (mean %/item), current drinkers	0.9	4.2	2.4	2.5	7.6	10.7	8.9
Problems score, all adults	0.7	1.9	0.9	0.2	0.5	4.3	2.0
Guilt/problem ratio	1.1	0.5	4.6	0	2.1	1.2	0.4
GENDER RATIOS							
Problems score, current drinkers	5.6	3.0	2.7	2.7	1.7	2.1	1.0
Problems score, all adults	6.7	4.2	4.2	19.5	8.4	2.6	1.9

abstainers among women means that the gender ratio becomes higher everywhere when scores are computed on a base including the abstainers. Even on a base of all adults, the Ugandan sample stands out in both genders with a higher rate of reported problems than elsewhere, with Costa Rican males also showing a relatively high rate. On a population basis, only in Uganda does the alcohol problem score for females reach above 2%.

As noted above, we included the item on feelings of guilt or remorse after drinking in the present analysis with the idea of examining the extent to which disapproval of problematic drinking is internalized in the different populations and subgroups. Table 3 shows that guilt or remorse after drinking was particularly common among Indian drinkers of both genders, and also fairly common among Ugandan and Brazilian male and female drinkers and among Sri Lankan male drinkers. A guilt/problem score ratio was computed and is shown in the third row for each gender in Table 4. On this basis, Indian and Brazilian problematic drinkers of both genders stand out as having relatively high guilt/problem ratios, with Sri Lankan males also relatively high. In Nigeria and Costa Rica, on the other hand, the guilt/problem ratio was relatively low in both genders, and in Uganda for males. The results of this analysis do not suggest that Ugandans might be specially sensitive to the existence of alcohol problems, which might have resulted in a lower threshold for reporting problems.

PROBLEM SCORES AND THE GUILT/PROBLEM RATIO BY GENDER AND AGE

In Table 5 we extend the analysis of the problem score to the question of variations by age. Argentinian males show the pattern which is commonly found in studies in the U.S. (Hilton, 1991) and some other developed countries (though not all): the highest rate of alcohol-related problems in young adulthood, a substantial drop-off after that, and a further drop-off in older age. Costa Rican females also show this pattern, but elsewhere in the table the patterns are diverse. Among Ugandan male drinkers, the highest rate is found in the middle age group, while among Ugandan females and Indians and Nigerians of both genders the oldest age group reports the highest rate. The findings are a strong caution that, considered in a global frame, patterns by age and gender differ considerably.

Table 5 also shows results by gender and age for the guilt/problem ratio described in the previous section. The base numbers are often small, making any ratio rather unstable; the Brazilian, Sri Lankan and Indian female figure should be treated with special caution. Looking at the other samples, there is some evidence that the guilt/problem ratio declines with age among Argentinian and Nigerian male drinkers, but this does not seem to be a general tendency.

TABLE 5.   **Problem scores among current drinkers and guilt/problem ratio, by gender and age, and gender ratios on drinking problem rates for drinkers, by age, among those aged 18-65 in seven developing countries, GENACIS surveys**
* denominator of ratio is 0

Age	Argentina	Costa Rica	Brazil	Sri Lanka	India	Uganda	Nigeria
MALE DRINKERS - problem score (mean % per item)							
Age <30	8.1	17.6	8.7	6.6	14.1	26.5	6.3
30-49	4.4	8.8	7.1	7.3	14.8	28.6	8.7
50+	1.6	10.6	2.5	5.6	20.6	20.8	11.5
FEMALE DRINKERS - problem score							
Age <30	1.3	6.6	4.9	0	7.3	13.6	4.5
30-49	0.2	3.3	1.2	3.7	8.1	13.6	9.1
50+	1.2	0.4	1.2	2.1	12.2	17.6	13.2
MALE DRINKERS - guilt/problem ratio							
Age <30	1.7	0.6	2.7	1.0	2.2	0.6	1.2
30-49	0.7	0.7	1.4	1.6	2.0	0.6	1.0
50+	0	0.8	0	3.0	1.9	0.7	0.6
FEMALE DRINKERS - guilt/problem ratio							
Age <30	1.2	0.7	2.6	*	2.9	1.3	0
30-49	3.0	0.3	6.4	0	1.0	1.0	0.8
50+	0	0	9.3	0	1.6	1.3	0.2
GENDER RATIO - problems score, current drinkers							
Age <30	6.2	2.7	1.8	*	1.9	1.9	1.4
30-49	22.0	2.7	5.9	2.0	1.8	2.1	1.0
50+	1.3	26.5	2.1	2.7	1.7	1.2	0.9

The last three rows in table 5 show the gender ratio on the problems score by age. Again, low underlying rates and Ns mean that the results must be treated with caution. Nigeria shows a tendency for the gender ratio to decline with increasing age, but this does not seem to be a general pattern in the other samples.

CONCLUSION

On a population basis, rates of self-reported alcohol problems are relatively low among women in all the societies studied, although among women in the two African societies studied, and particularly in Uganda, the rates reported were higher than elsewhere. Part of the explanation for the low rates is the relatively high rate of abstinence among women in all the societies studied except Argentina. But even on a base of current drinkers, women reported fewer problems than men from their own drinking in all samples except Nigeria, where the rates among drinkers were equal.

There was considerable diversity in the patterning of alcohol problems by age. One or more examples could be found of the highest rate occurring in each of the three age groups studied. Thus the pattern found in U.S. and some other studies, of a fall in alcohol problem rates in the late 20s and another in or after the 50s, should not be assumed to hold elsewhere. Among African and Indian drinkers, indeed, there was evidence of an increase in problem rates with increasing age.

Ugandan drinkers, both men and women, showed especially high rates of alcohol problems, a finding which in general fits the data from other sources showing a high rate of per-capita alcohol consumption and relatively hazardous drinking patterns. On a total-population basis, the problem rates of Costa Rican men also stood out, and Nigerian women stood out in comparison to other women.

The general conclusion to be drawn from alcohol's relatively high ranking as a risk factor for death and disability (Ezzati et al., 2002; Room et al., 2005) is that a major effort to strengthen alcohol policies is needed on a global basis. The need is particularly strong, it would seem, in some of the countries included in the present analysis.

REFERENCES

Babor, T., Caetano, R., Casswell, S., Edwards, G., Giesbrecht, N., Graham, K., Grube, J., Gruenewald, P., Hill, L., Holder, H., Homel, R., Österberg, E., Rehm, J., Room, R., & Rossow, I. (2003). *Alcohol: No Ordinary Commodity – Research and Public Policy.* Oxford, etc.: Oxford University Press.

Demers, A., Room, R., & Bourgault, C. (eds., 2001). *Surveys of Drinking Patterns and Problems in Seven Developing Countries.* Geneva: World Health Organization, Department of Mental Health and Substance Dependence, WHO/MSD/MSB/01.2.

Ezzati, M., Lopez, A.D., Rodgers, A., Vander Hoorn, S., Murray, C.J.L., & the Comparative Risk Assessment Collaborating Group (2002) Selected major risk factors and global and regional burden of disease. *The Lancet* **360**, 1347-1360.

Hilton, M.E. (1991) The demographic distribution of drinking problems in 1984. In: W.B. Clark & M.E. Hilton, eds. *Alcohol in America: Drinking Practices and Problems* (pp. 87-101). Albany: State University of New York Press.

Rehm, J., Monteiro, M., Room, R., Gmel, G., Jernigan, D., Frick, U., & Graham, K. (2001). Steps towards constructing a global comparative risk analysis for alcohol consumption: determining indicators and empirical weights for patterns of drinking, deciding about theoretical minimum, and dealing with different consequences. *European Addiction Research* **7**, 138-147.

Rehm, J., Room, R., Monteiro, M., Gmel, G., Graham, K., Rehn, N., Sempos, C.T., Frick, U., & Jernigan, D. (2004). Alcohol. In: M. Ezzati, A.D. Lopez, A. Rodgers, & C.J.L. Murray, eds., *Comparative Quantification of Health Risks: Global and Regional Burden of Disease Attributable to Selected Major Risk Factors.* Volume 1 (pp. 959-1108). Geneva: World Health Organization.

Roizen, R. (1988). Cultural control of drinking by universal moderation or differential access. Presented at the annual meeting of the Society for Cross-Cultural Studies, El Paso, Texas, August. http://www.roizen.com/ron/elpaso.htm

Room, R., Jernigan, D., Carlini-Marlatt, B., Gureje, O., Mäkelä, K., Marshall, M., Medina-Mora, M.E., Monteiro, M., Parry, C., Partanen, J., Riley, L., & Saxena, S. (2002). *Alcohol and Developing Societies: A Public Health Approach.* Helsinki: Finnish Foundation for Alcohol Studies & Geneva: World Health Organization.

Room, R. (2005). Alcohol policy: issues and challenges for the W.H.O. European Region. Presented at a WHO-Euro meeting on Alcohol Policy in the WHO European Region, Stora Brännbo, Sigtuna, Sweden, 13-15 April.

Room, R., Babor, T., & Rehm, J. (2005). Alcohol and public health: a review. *The Lancet* **365**:519-530.

WHO (2004). *Global Status Report: Alcohol Policy.* Geneva: World Health Organization, Department of Mental Health and Substance Abuse.

AUTHORS

VICTOR ADETULA

Dr Adetula is Associate Professor of political science at the University of Jos, Nigeria, with a wide range of experience in development work. He has conducted research and published articles, book chapters and monographs on broad issues of development in Nigeria, Africa and Europe.

JULIO BEJARANO

A researcher at Fundación Vida y Sociedad and the Instituto sobre Alcoholismo y Farmacodependencia, Costa Rica, Bejarano is also a professor of Psychology at Universidad Estatal a Distancia and at the Iberoamerican Master's Degree Program on Drug Dependence. He has authored several books and papers on alcohol and other drug epidemiology.

VIVEK BENEGAL

Dr Benegal is Associate Professor of psychiatry at the Deaddiction Centre at the National Institute of Mental Health and Neuro-Sciences (NIMHANS), Bangalore, India, a regional centre for substance abuse studies for southern India. His areas of research interest are the epidemiology of alcohol use disorders in India, genetics and neurobiology of alcoholism and the social and political history of alcohol in the Indian sub-continent. His recent work has focused on the prevalence of undocumented alcohol consumption, the association between alcohol and injuries in India and the study of high risk markers of susceptibility to alcoholism.

PRABHA S.CHANDRA

Dr Chandra is Additional Professor of Psychiatry at NIMHANS, an executive member of the Women's Section of the World Psychiatric Association, and a member of the Advisory group on Behavioral Research in HIV/AIDS of the Indian Council of Medical Research and the National AIDS Control Organization (Governemnt of India). Her main areas of interest are: women's mental health, psychosocial aspects of HIV/AIDS, HIV related risk among different populations including substance users.

ZUBAIRU KWAMBO DAGONA

Dagona is a Senior Lecturer and clinical psychologist with the Department of General and Applied Psychology, University of Jos, Nigeria. His areas of research interest include child clinical psychology, psychology of substance use and abuse, and traffic psychology.

ANA DURAND

A research assistant for Dr. Romero mainly in the study on addiction problems in female prisoners, Durand obtained her bachelor's degree in psychology at the National Autonomous University of Mexico. She also has a diploma in Eating Disorders and Addictions and currently studying for her master's degree in psychotherapy. Her research interests are related to sexual abuse and substance abuse in women.

TRICIA M. F . FLORIPES

A Social worker in the Department of Neurology and Psychiatry of Botucatu Medical School, University of São Paulo State (Universidade Estadual Paulista, Floripes has a FAPESP fellowship and her main interest is in treatment and prevention of alcohol abuse.

G. GURURAJ

Dr Gururaj is Professor and Head of the Department of Epidemiology (a WHO Collaborating Centre for injury prevention and safety promotion) at the National Institute of Mental Health and Neuro-Sciences, Bangalore, India. His primary interests are injury epidemiology, prevention and control, and psychiatric epidemiology. He is actively involved in translation of research to policies and programmes at local and national levels. He is a member of several technical committees and has several publications to his credit.

ANDREA M. HEGEDUS

Research Assistant Professor in the Department of Psychiatry at the University of Michigan, An Arbor, USA, Dr Hegedus' interests include alcohol and associated consequences with a special interest in gender issues.

SIRI HETTIGE

Senior Professor of Sociology at the University of Colombo, Dr Hettige's research and writing on alcohol issues spread over the last two decades. He has publicly advocated the need for a comprehensive national policy on alcohol in Sri Lanka, a goal yet to be achieved. He has B.A. and B.Phil. degrees in sociology from the University of Colombo and a Ph.D. degree in Social Anthropology from Monash University, Australia.

AKANIDOMO K. J. IBANGA

Ibanga is Senior Lecturer in the Department of Psychology University of Jos, Jos, Nigeria, and deputy director, Centre for Research and

Information on Substance Abuse (CRISA), Jos. He has been actively engaged in research and writing on alcohol and other drugs with several publications and book chapters in this area.

HARUNA KARICK

Karick is a Lecturer in clinical psychology with the Department of General and Applied Psychology of the University of Jos, Jos, Nigeria. His research interests include substance abuse and stress management.

FLORENCE KERR-CORRÊA

Dr Kerr-Corrêa is a Professor of Psychiatry at the Department of Neurology and Psychiatry of Botucatu Medical School, University of São Paulo State (Universidade Estadual Paulista), UNESP Brazil. She is responsible for the UNESP Treatment and Prevention Program on Alcohol and Drug Abuse and has a special interest in gender issues concerning alcohol/drug abuse and affective disorders.

LIGIA R. S. KERR-PONTES

Associate Professor of Epidemiology in the Department of Epidemiology at the Department of Community Health of the Federal University of Ceará, her primary areas of work are in HIV and leprosy. She is a consultant on STD and AIDS Programme of the Brazilian Ministry of Health and of the D. Libânia National Reference Centre of Leprosy.

NAZARIUS TUMWESIGYE MBONA

A Lecturer in the Department of Biostatistics and Epidemiology at the Institute of Public Health, Makerere University, Kampala, Uganda, Mbona is currently on study leave pursuing a doctoral degree at the University of Southampton, UK. He has a Mater of Arts degree in demography from Makerere University and a Master of Science degree in medical statistics from the London School of Hygiene and Tropical Medicine (LSHTM). His research interests include dynamics of condom use and sexual abstinence, general sexual and reproductive health, and how alcohol use might be linked to sexual activity and condom use.

MA. ELENA MEDINA-MORA

Professor in the Faculty of Medicine and Faculty of Psychology at the National Autonomous University of Mexico and director of Epidemiological and Psychosocial Research at the National Institute of Psychiatry, Medina-Mora is a pioneer in epidemiological studies on addictions in Mexico and has been in charge of the National Addictions Survey that has provided fundamental information for health policies in Mexico in relation to addiction problems. She has served in many advisory committees of the World Health Organization.

MYRIAM MUNNE

Psychologist with postgraduate training in alcohol and drugs research at the University of Buenos Aires, Argentina, Munne has worked as a researcher in NGOs, Ministry of Justice, and the National Council of Youth and Family of Argentina and collaborated in prevention programmes on substance abuse at the University of Buenos Aires. She was Principal Investigator of the GENACIS study in Argentina, and study leader for Argentina in the Multicentric Study on Gender, Alcohol and Harm of Alcohol and Drug Abuse at the Pan American Health Organization (PAHO).

PRATIMA MURTHY

Murthy is Additional Professor of psychiatry at the National Institute of Mental Health and Neuro Sciences, Bangalore, India, where she completed her psychiatric training. She has been a consultant to the International Labour Organization and the United Nations Office on Drugs and Crime. She has authored monographs on women and substance use in India and community based drug rehabilitation and workplace prevention.

MADHABIKA B. NAYAK

Dr Nayak is Associate Scientist at the Alcohol Research Group, Public Health Institute in Berkeley, California. Her research, clinical, and teaching interests pertain to health issues, including interpersonal violence and cultural factors that affect both drinking and health. Her recent work has focused on problematic and risky drinking and relationships among alcohol use, interpersonal violence, and health.

ISIDORE S. OBOT

Currently a Scientist in the Department of Mental Health and Substance Abuse at the World Health Organization, Geneva, Switzerland, Dr Obot's career in the addictions field and as a teacher of psychology in Nigeria and the USA spans over twenty years. He is founding Editor-in-chief of the *African Journal of Drug and Alcohol Studies* and Assistant Editor of *Addiction*. His research interests are in substance use epidemiology and prevention.

Ochinya Ojiji

Dr Ojiji is a social psychologist and assistant director at the Centre for Peace and Conflict Resolution in Abuja, Nigeria. He was formerly a lecturer in the Department of Psychology at the University of Jos, and the University of Uyo, Nigeria.

Dharmadasa Paranagama

A statistician and a demographer in training, he functioned as the research officer for the GENACIS study in Sri Lanka is. Paranagama has a B. A. degree in anthropology from the University of Vidyodaya, Sri Lanka, a Diploma in Population Studies from University of Colombo and a Master of Arts degree in demography from the Australian National University.

Rogers Kasirye

Director of the Uganda Youth Development Link (UYDEL), an organization that runs prevention and counseling programmes for young people in Uganda, Kasirye was the first winner of the Vienna Civil Society Award of the United nations Office on Drugs and Crime in 1999. He has been an investigator in alcohol related studies in Uganda.

Martha Romero

Dr Romero obtained her clinical psychology degree at the Universidad Iberoamericana, Mexico City and a Master's degree in clinical psychology at the National Autonomous University of Mexico. She has been working since 1985 at the National Institute of Psychiatry as a researcher. Her main research interests have been in qualitative research and the study of addictions in women.

Robin Room

Robin Room is Professor and Director of the Centre for Social Research on Alcohol and Drugs at Stockholm University, Stockholm, Sweden. His research focus has been on epidemiological, social and cultural studies of alcohol, but he has also done work in other areas of drug and gambling problems. He is a coauthor of *Alcohol in Developing Societies: A Public Health Approach* (2002) and a coeditor of *Surveys of Drinking Patterns and Problems in Seven Developing Countries* (2001).

Alessandra F. Sanches

Social worker in the Department of Neurology and Psychiatry of University of Sao Paulo (Unesp) at Botucatu Medical School, she completed a Fapesp

(Fundação do Amparo à Pesquisa do Estado de São Paulo) fellowship. Her primary interest is in treatment and prevention of alcohol abuse.

KLARA HRADILOVA SELIN

Klara H. Selin is a PhD student in sociology at the Centre for Social Research on Alcohol and Drugs at Stockholm University, Stockholm, Sweden. Her main research area is epidemiological studies on drinking behaviour, with a special interest in family matters, informal social control and harm from drinking to a third party.

LUZIA A. TRINCA

Trinca is Associate Professor of Statistics in the Department of Biostatistics, Biosciences Institute, UNESP, Sao Paulo, Brazil. She has considerable experience working in addiction research.

ADRIANA M. TUCCI

Psychologist with a Master's degree in Mental Health and doctoral student in the Department of Psychobiology, São Paulo Federal University (UNIFESP) where she is working on child abuse and its co-occurrence with alcohol and drug abuse.

JORGE VILLATORO

Social researcher at the Direction of Epidemiological and Social Research at the National Institute of Psychiatry. He has been in charge of developing the Student Survey on Addictions that provides information for Mexico City and also at the national level. He teaches statistics at the Master's and Doctorate degree programmes on public and mental health areas.

RICHARD W. WILSNACK

Dr Wilsnack is Professor in the Department of Clinical Neuroscience, University of North Dakota School of Medicine and Health Sciences and editor (with Sharon Wilsnack) of the book *Gender and Alcohol: Individual and Social Perspectives* (Rutgers Center of Alcohol Studies, 1997). He has served as a consultant on alcohol research for the National Institute on Alcohol Abuse and Alcoholism and for the Robert Wood Johnson Foundation, and as chair of the Drinking and Drugs Division of the Society for the Study of Social Problems. His current research interests are in (1) how biology and culture combine to create gender differences in alcohol use, (2) how men and women drink as couples, and (3) how women's drinking patterns change across their lifespans.

Sharon Carlson Wilsnack

Chester Fritz Distinguished Professor in the Department of Clinical Neuroscience, University of North Dakota School of Medicine and Health Sciences, she is co-editor with Linda Beckman of the volume *Alcohol Problems in Women: Antecedents, Consequences, and Intervention* (New York: Guilford Press, 1984) and with Richard Wilsnack of *Gender and Alcohol: Individual and Social Perspectives* (Rutgers Center of Alcohol Studies, 1997). Sharon Wilsnack is a Fellow of the American Psychological Association and has served in numerous boards and advisory groups, including as a member of the National Advisory Committee, White House Office of National Drug Control Policy.